Social Media in Medicine

The use of social media around the world has exploded in recent years, with the number of monthly active users of Facebook and Twitter estimated to be one billion and one quarter billion, respectively. Physicians and medical trainees are among the users of social media, raising questions of how Facebook, Twitter, and other novel online tools may best be harnessed to further medical research, patient care, and educational pursuits. Because social media enables an immediate exchange of information and ideas around shared areas of interest, it has fostered communication and collaboration among a global network of researchers, clinicians, patients, and learners. *Social Media in Medicine* reviews a range of topics, from research ethics to medical education, and includes personal reflections by clinicians and learners that represent diverse opinions about the role of social media in medicine. This book is relevant to all health-care stakeholders and will hopefully encourage ideas and questions to generate more research into the use of social media in medical research, patient care, and education. This book was originally published as a special issue of the *International Review of Psychiatry*.

Margaret S. Chisolm is an Associate Professor and the Vice Chair for Education in the Department of Psychiatry and Behavioral Sciences at Johns Hopkins University, Baltimore, MD, USA. She writes about substance use, humanistic practice, and medical education; and is a Miller-Coulson Academy of Clinical Excellence member, an Arnold P. Gold Foundation Humanism Scholar, and 2014 Johns Hopkins University Alumni Association Excellence in Teaching Award recipient. @whole_patients

Social Media in Medicine

Edited by
Margaret S. Chisolm

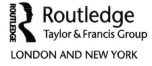

Routledge
Taylor & Francis Group

LONDON AND NEW YORK

First published 2016 by Routledge

2 Park Square, Milton Park, Abingdon, Oxfordshire OX14 4RN
711 Third Avenue, New York, NY 10017

Routledge is an imprint of the Taylor & Francis Group, an informa business

First issued in paperback 2018

British Library Cataloguing in Publication Data
A catalogue record for this book is available from the British Library

ISBN 13: 978-1-138-66538-5 (hbk)
ISBN 13: 978-0-367-02278-5 (pbk)

Typeset in Plantin
by diacriTech, Chennai

Publisher's Note
The publisher accepts responsibility for any inconsistencies that may have arisen
during the conversion of this book from journal articles to book chapters, namely
the possible inclusion of journal terminology.

Disclaimer
Every effort has been made to contact copyright holders for their permission to
reprint material in this book. The publishers would be grateful to hear from any
copyright holder who is not here acknowledged and will undertake to rectify any
errors or omissions in future editions of this book.

Contents

Citation Information

The chapters in this book were originally published in the *International Review of Psychiatry*, volume 27, issue 2 (April 2015). When citing this material, please use the original page numbering for each article, as follows:

CITATION INFORMATION

Chapter 8
Social media, medicine and the modern journal club
Joel M. Topf and Swapnil Hiremath
International Review of Psychiatry, volume 27, issue 2 (April 2015) pp. 147–154

Chapter 9
A personal reflection on social media in medicine: I stand, no wiser than before
John Weiner
International Review of Psychiatry, volume 27, issue 2 (April 2015) pp. 155–160

Chapter 10
Personal reflections on exploring social media in medicine
Brent Thoma
International Review of Psychiatry, volume 27, issue 2 (April 2015) pp. 161–166

Chapter 11
My three shrinks: Personal stories of social media exploration
Steve Daviss, Annette Hanson and Dinah Miller
International Review of Psychiatry, volume 27, issue 2 (April 2015) pp. 167–173

For any permission-related enquiries please visit:
http://www.tandfonline.com/page/help/permissions

Notes on Contributors

Ashish Atreja is an Assistant Professor and the Director of Sinai AppLab in the Division of Gastroenterology and Chief Technology Innovation and Engagement Officer (C-TIE) in the Department of Medicine at the Icahn School of Medicine at Mount Sinai. His work supports the development of point-of-care multi-centric registries, registries, quality improvement dashboards, and development and evaluation. @atreja

Margaret S. Chisolm is an Associate Professor and the Vice Chair for Education in the Department of Psychiatry and Behavioral Sciences at Johns Hopkins University, Baltimore, MD, USA. She writes about substance use, humanistic practice, and medical education; and is a Miller-Coulson Academy of Clinical Excellence member, an Arnold P. Gold Foundation Humanism Scholar, and 2014 Johns Hopkins University Alumni Association Excellence in Teaching Award recipient. @whole_patients

Katherine C. Chretien is the Assistant Dean for Student Affairs and an Associate Professor of Medicine at George Washington University, Washington, DC, USA, and the Chief of the Hospitalist Section at the Washington DC Veterans Affairs Medical Center. Her academic focus has been on the intersection of social media in medicine and professionalism. @MotherinMed

Steve Daviss is the Chief Medical Information Officer at M3 Information; the developer of the multidimensional mental health assessment tool for primary care, M3 Checklist; double-boarded in Psychiatry and in Psychosomatic Medicine, with a focus on quality measures and health information technology; a clinical assistant professor at University of Maryland School of Medicine; recent past Chairman of the Department of Psychiatry at University of Maryland Baltimore Washington Medical Center; and the founding President at FUSE Health Strategies. He chairs the APA Committee on Mental Health Information Technology and serves on numerous committees and boards addressing quality, policy, informatics, and standards in healthcare. @HITshrink.

Matthew DeCamp is an Assistant Professor of Medicine, based in the Berman Institute of Bioethics and Division of General Internal Medicine, at Johns Hopkins University, Baltimore, MD, USA. His research interests include social media and medical professionalism, ethics and patient engagement in health care reform, and global health. @MattDeCamp1

Alexander M. Djuricich is the Education Editor for the New England Journal of Medicine Group. His research interests include internal medicine, pediatrics, adolescent medicine, and quality improvement. @MedPedsDoctor

Yolanda Evans is a member of the Division of Adolescent Medicine at Seattle Children's Hospital, WA, USA, and an Assistant Professor of Pediatrics at the School of Medicine, University of Washington, Seattle, WA, USA. @akcoco

Jason Frank is the Director, Specialty Education, Strategy and Standards in the Office of Specialty Education at the Royal College of Physicians and Surgeons of Canada, as well as the Vice-Chair, Education and the Director of Educational Research & Development in the Department of Emergency Medicine, University of Ottawa, Canada. @drjfrank

Annette Hanson is the Director of the Forensic Psychiatry Fellowship at the University of Maryland, College Park, MD, USA. She has more than 20 years of experience as a correctional psychiatrist, and has cared for pre-trial detainees and sentenced offenders at all levels of security. @ClinkShrink

NOTES ON CONTRIBUTORS

Swapnil Hiremath is an Assistant Professor in the Faculty of Medicine at the University of Ottawa, Canada, and an Associate Investigator in the Clinical Epidemiology Program at the Ottawa Hospital Research Institute. His research interests include clinical outcomes research in hypertension, vascular access, and acute kidney injury. @hswapnil

Alireza Jalali is the Teaching Chair and a Distinguished Teacher of the Faculty of Medicine at the University of Ottawa, Canada. His research interests include e-learning, innovations in teaching and anatomy. @ARJalali

Terry Kind is an Associate Professor of Pediatrics and the Assistant Dean for Clinical Education at George Washington University and a primary care pediatrician at Children's National in Washington, DC, USA. Her professional interests include medical education, reflective practice, lifelong learning, social media, and professionalism. @Kind4Kids

Natalie T. Lafferty heads the Centre for Technology and Innovation in Learning at the University of Dundee, Dundee, UK, and teaches in the School of Medicine. Her research interests include the use of social technologies to support open educational practice, engaging students as producers of learning, and the innovative use of technology to enhance learning. @nlafferty

Annalisa Manca is an educationalist and advisor working in medical/health-care education at both national and international level. Based at the School of Medicine in the University of Dundee, Dundee, UK, she specializes in the use of emerging, social technologies to support health-care education and continuing professional development. Her research interests focus on how social technologies can be employed to facilitate students' engagement and learning, staff development, and compassionate care. @AnnalisaManca

Neil Mehta is a Staff Physician at the Cleveland Clinic, Cleveland, OH, USA. He is also the Assistant Dean for Education Informatics and Technology and an Associate Professor of Medicine at the Cleveland Clinic Lerner College of Medicine at Case Western Reserve University and the Director of the Center for Technology-enhanced Knowledge and Instruction (cTEKI), Cleveland, OH, USA. His speciality interests include chronic disease management, diagnostic internal medicine, and the management of patients with multiple complex problems. @Neil_Mehta

Dinah Miller is a psychiatrist and writer working in Baltimore, MD, USA. @shrinkrapdinah

Jonathan Sherbino is an Associate Professor in the Division of Emergency Medicine at McMaster University, Hamilton, Canada. He is also an emergency physician and trauma team leader in Hamilton. He is a clinician-educator with the Royal College of Physicians and Surgeons of Canada. @sherbino

Stephanie Sutherland is currently based in the Faculty of Medicine at the University of Ottawa, Canada. @StephanieSuthe1

Brent Thoma is a Clinical Assistant Professor in the College of Medicine at the University of Saskatchewan, Saskatoon, Canada. In 2015, he was awarded the Robert Maudsley Fellowship for Studies in Medical Education at the Royal College of Physicians and Surgeons of Canada. @Brent_Thoma

Joel M. Topf is a clinical nephrologist based in Detriot, MI, USA. He is an assistant clinical professor at Oakland University William Beaumont School of Medicine in Rochester, MI, USA. @kidney_boy

Matthew G. Tuck is an Assistant Professor of Medicine at George Washington University, Washington, DC, USA, and the Associate Site Program Director for the residency programs at the Washington DC Veterans Affairs Medical Center. His major research interests include anemia, thrombosis, evidence-based medicine, and medical education.

John Weiner is a consultant physician in Melbourne, Australia. His website AllergyNet Australia, launched in January 1998, is archived by the National Library of Australia as the oldest continuous medical blog in the world. He has co-authored several papers on social media in education with the Medical Education Research and Quality Unit at Monash University, Melbourne, Australia. @AllergyNet

Janine E. Zee-Cheng is a pediatric intensivist currently practicing in Wisconsin. @JanineZeeCheng

Social media in medicine: The volume that Twitter built

The use of social media around the world has exploded in recent years, with the number of monthly active users of Facebook and Twitter estimated to be one billion and one quarter billion, respectively (Facebook, 2014; Twitter, 2015). Healthcare professionals and learners are among the users of social media, raising questions of how Facebook, Twitter, and other novel online tools may best be harnessed to further medicine's research, patient care, and educational goals. Because social media enables an immediate exchange of information and ideas around shared areas of interest, it has fostered communication and collaboration among a global network of scientific investigators, clinicians, patients, and learners. Psychiatry has been a relatively late adopter of social media compared to other medical specialities, perhaps due – in part – to heightened concerns regarding patient confidentiality and clinician privacy. This social media in medicine issue of the *International Review of Psychiatry* will explore these and other topics relevant not only to psychiatrists, but all of all healthcare stakeholders.

Not only is this the first ever volume of the *International Review of Psychiatry* whose content is focused on social media, but this is also the first volume of this journal developed almost entirely via social media. All of the articles in this issue, with the exception of two, were authored by individuals I first encountered on Twitter. Thus, this is truly the first volume of the *International Review of Psychiatry* that Twitter built.

The papers in this issue focus on a spectrum of topics of interest both to academic and non-academic scientific investigators, clinicians, educators, and trainees, as well as patients. The goal is to critically review the available evidence regarding an array of topics, ranging from research ethics to educational endeavours. The issue also includes several personal reflections by an experienced group of clinicians and learners, who have diverse opinions regarding the value of social media in medicine.

This volume begins with an exploration of the use of social media in research. Natalie Lafferty and Annalisa Manca from the University of Dundee review the types of social media tools currently being used in research, how these tools are being used, and both the benefits and challenges of their use. The use of social media in research is an area of intense innovation, with many methodological approaches still in the process of being tested. Nevertheless, this review will be of use to scientific investigators, including psychiatrists, who are interested in developing a more informed approach to the use of social media in research. A related topic is addressed by Matthew DeCamp from the Johns Hopkins University Berman Institute of Bioethics and School of Medicine who reviews the major ethical issues arising from social media use in research, public health, mobile health applications, and global health. As social media tools continue to emerge, understanding the relevant ethical issues will be critical to the success of healthcare applications while preserving medicine's core value as a public trust. Public good also plays a role in online professionalism, as described by Katherine Chretien and Matthew Tuck from the George Washington University School of Medicine and Health Services. An area of keen interest to psychiatrists, they characterize the methodological approaches of the social media and professionalism studies to date, with an eye to enhancing future research in this important area.

Online professionalism is essential given social media's inherently public nature. Such open discourse has its advantages, especially to patients. Social media can be used to encourage conversations about specific disorders and their treatment and to offer support for patients via public awareness campaigns, as well as online social groups. Neil Mehta of Cleveland Clinic Lerner College of Medicine of Case Western Reserve University and Ashish Atreja of Icahn School of Medicine at Mount Sinai provide an overview of online support groups, their unique challenges, and how they can complement traditional healthcare delivery models.

A major emphasis of this issue is on the use of social media in medical education. Social media – integrated into training at the undergraduate, graduate, and continuing medical education levels – has the potential to enhance lifelong learning. Terry Kind of George Washington University School of Medicine and Health Sciences and Yolanda Evans of University of Washington School of Medicine present examples from the peer-reviewed literature of how the use of social media in the training of medical and other healthcare students can provide them the skills they will need for lifelong learning. Medical conferences also represent an opportunity to incorporate social media into lifelong learning, as described by Alexander Djuricich and Janine Zee-Chang of Indiana University School of Medicine. The authors focus on how Twitter can be used by physicians and other healthcare providers at local, regional, national, and international conferences to expand on the formal education provided in these venues. Using a detailed content analysis of the Twitter transcript from one international conference, Alireza Jalali and Stephanie Sutherland of University of Ottawa and Jonathan Sherbino and Jason Frank of the Royal College of Physicians and Surgeons of Canada, suggest several mechanisms by which this social media tool is able to enhance the educational value of academic conferences.

The final section of the issue features more personal viewpoints regarding social media in medicine. First, Joel Topf of the Oakland University William Beaumont School of Medicine and Swapnil Hiremath of the University of Ottawa offer an engaging history of medical education media (from print to social) to introduce the story of their creation of a Twitter-based nephrology journal club. Next, Steve Daviss and Annette Hanson of the University of Maryland School of Medicine and Dinah Miller of the Johns Hopkins University School of Medicine share how they have maintained a blog since 2006, produced over 65 audio podcasts, and participated in other forms of social media, including Twitter. The authors each provide a narrative account of his/her personal social media journey: Daviss as an advocate for our profession, Hanson as a medical educator, and Miller as a patient advocate. John Weiner of the Monash University School of Public Health and Preventive Medicine provides an equally deeply informed, but different, perspective. The author, who is 67

years old and has maintained a medical blog since 1998, is considered a pioneer in the field of social media in medicine. Yet he remains 'restless and confused' on the topic, and in his reflection raises a number of compelling questions about the impact of these tools on clinical excellence and medical education, which are to be 'answered in the next generation.' This leads to the final paper in the issue, by Brent Thoma of the University of Saskatchewan, who describes how, as an emergency medicine resident, he created a blog – at first using a pseudonym – as a way of gingerly exploring social media. Thoma is now one of the leading scholars in the field of social media in medicine and has clearly found his voice.

It is hoped that the papers included in this special issue convey the excitement of participating in this cutting-edge field, as well as some of the challenges. These papers will hopefully encourage ideas and questions and inspire more research into the use of social media in all aspects of medicine: research, patient care, and education. I am grateful to the authors and reviewers for the enormous time and energy devoted to this issue and thank the editors for the invitation to produce such a timely volume.

Margaret S. Chisolm
Department of Psychiatry and Behavioral Sciences
Johns Hopkins University School of Medicine
Baltimore, Maryland, USA

Declaration of interest: The authors report no conflicts of interest. The authors alone are responsible for the content and writing of the paper.

References

Facebook.(2014). Facebook Newsroom. Retrieved 30 April 2014 from http://newsroom.fb.com/company-info/ (Facebook, December 31, 2014; accessed today 3/23/15)

Twitter. (2014). About Twitter. Retrieved 30 April 2014 from https://about.twitter.com/company (Twitter, 2015, accessed today 3/23/15)

Perspectives on social media in and as research: A synthetic review

NATALIE T. LAFFERTY[1] & ANNALISA MANCA[2]

[1]*Library and Learning Centre, Centre for Technology and Innovation in Learning, University of Dundee, Dundee, UK*
[2]*Medical Education Institute, School of Medicine, University of Dundee, Ninewells Hospital & Medical School, UK.*

Abstract

With the growth of social media use in both the private and public spheres, researchers are currently exploring the new opportunities and practices offered by these tools in the research lifecycle. This area is still in its infancy: As methodological approaches and methods are being tested – mainly through pragmatic and exploratory approaches – practices are being shaped and negotiated by the actors involved in research. A further element of complexity is added by the ambivalent status of social media within research activities. They can be both a tool – for recruitment, data collection, analysis – and data – as what constitutes the corpus to be analysed – both in an observational and interactive domain. This synthetic analysis of the literature is aimed at identifying how social media are currently being used in research and how they fit into the research lifecycle. We identify and discuss emerging evidence and trends in the adoption of social media in research, which can be used and applied by psychiatry research practitioners as a framework to inform the development of a personalized research network and social media strategy in research.

Introduction

The birth of the 'read, write web' and 'Web 2.0' technologies has seen a proliferation of social media (SoMe) tools providing new opportunities for connecting and communicating, and for creating and sharing information. Whilst many of these tools and technologies were not developed with a specific intention to support research or education, as individuals have used these tools they have applied and made use of them in their professional lives. SoMe is providing new opportunities and there is a sense of being on the cusp of a new wave in research (Bartling & Friesike, 2014) that challenges traditional modes of research dissemination and offers new opportunities for engaging with patients and the public at large.

While SoMe have been identified as having the potential to change the way researchers work, collaborate and communicate (Archibald & Clark, 2014; Das et al., 2014; Grosseck & Holotescu, 2011; Kapp et al., 2013; Ovadia, 2009) both amongst themselves and with participants and the public, the actual use of SoMe in research is still in its infancy (O'Connor, 2013; van Osch & Coursaris, 2014). In this paper we review some of the emerging evidence and commentaries on the adoption and role of SoMe in research which may inform their further application in medical and healthcare research.

Objectives

This paper presents a synthetic literature review of published studies that used SoMe in any stage of the research cycle and studies or commentaries that addressed the topic of SoMe use in research. As such, we briefly summarize findings, opinions and discussion about the use of SoMe in research, including examples from psychiatry, and we discuss how the literature can be used to help researchers support the development of personalized research frameworks.

Through this synthetic analysis we attempt to answer the following research questions:

1. How is SoMe being used in current research?
2. What tools are being used and how?
3. How does SoMe fit into elements of the research lifecycle?
4. What are the perceived and evident benefits?
5. What are the main challenges that need to be addressed?

Methods

Three electronic databases (Taylor & Francis, Wiley and PubMed) were searched for papers containing the following keywords in the title or abstract: 'research AND social media OR twitter OR blog OR facebook OR microblog OR digital' between 2008 and 2014. Both authors then evaluated all the paper abstracts obtained for relevance and 56 out of 110 articles were identified and mutually agreed as suitable for inclusion in the review.

Due to their active engagement with SoMe in research and their familiarity with the issues involved, both authors felt the corpus needed to be further supplemented with papers, reports and guides that have informed our own use of SoMe in research and educational practice along with papers shared by our Twitter networks.

Due to the field of research analysed being rather immature, and therefore lacking methodological diversity (van Osch & Coursaris, 2014), we also included commentaries, books and reviews to take into account the wide range of current debate and theorization on this topic.

Preliminary considerations

We performed a preliminary thematic analysis of the selected literature, categorizing the studies according to the use or discussion of SoMe under the stages of the research lifecycle. Although research is an iterative and non-linear process (Nicholas & Rowlands, 2011), placing activities and tools into a four-step schematic approach was useful to identify the current trends in the use of SoMe in research. The four steps we examined were (1) the planning phase, including identifying the research topic, potential collaborators and initial review of the literature, (2) the development of the project, including a more detailed literature review, identifying underlying theories and methodologies, planning the project timeline, (3) the implementation of the research, i.e. enrolling participants, gathering data, and then analysis and interpretation of the data, and (4) dissemination of the research findings and engagement with the research community and the wider public.

The preliminary thematic analysis on the selected literature highlighted various complexities, as some research procedures clearly overlap several stages of the lifecycle in cases where SoMe is the source of research data. For this reason, after a brief discussion about SoMe in the research lifecycle, we report and discuss the role of 'SoMe as data' as a separate strand. We consider this using a model we adapted from Moreno et al. (2013), looking at SoMe as a source of data in two complementary dimensions. The aim of Moreno et al.'s paper was to provide a set of key ethical considerations for both researchers and institutional review boards (IRBs) or ethics committees called to review research projects involving SoMe. This highlights the various degrees of complexity surrounding this area, which touches researchers, participants and reviewers in different but connected strands.

Social media in the lifecycle of a research project

With levels of scepticism around the use of SoMe in research, a helpful way to consider their potential and application is to look at their role in relation to the research cycle. A major international study of the use of SoMe in research (Nicholas & Rowlands, 2011; Rowlands et al., 2011) indicates that SoMe are being used to identify research opportunities, support collaboration and to disseminate research findings. Procter et al. (2010) found that UK researchers valued the informality SoMe offered and that many were using at least one SoMe tool. Whilst researchers in health and medical sciences may not have the highest levels of adoption of SoMe (Procter et al., 2010) those that do use them find them of much more value in the research lifecycle than researchers from other disciplines (Nicholas & Rowlands, 2011). Emerging key perceived benefits of using SoME include the ability to connect with researchers across disciplines and geographic divides, and the ability to build and maintain research communities. These communities and networks are supported by platforms such as Facebook, LinkedIn, Google+, ResearchGate, Academia.edu, Mendeley, CiteULike and Twitter. In education the concepts of personal learning networks (PLN) and personal learning environments (PLE) have emerged (Attwell, 2007) to refer to the interaction between different agents and technologies involved in one's learning process. Similarly, as researchers increasingly adopt technology to support their own research, they are developing a personal research environment (PRE) and SoMe is facilitating connections across personal research networks (PRN). However, lack of appreciation of the benefits of SoMe together with perceived risks can pose a barrier for adoption (Davis, 1989). There are concerns over privacy, whilst the blurring of professional and personal online spaces and digital identities see work creeping into personal time (Cann et al., 2011). Other constraints include a sense of information overload, with an overwhelming number of tools to grasp and appreciate which ones can be trusted. Issues of trust in relation to integrity and quality of information also surround scholarly communication on SoMe platforms (Procter et al., 2010).

Planning

Developing a PRN takes time but brings benefits, increasing the connectedness of researchers, providing a platform to ask questions while also serving as a way of professionally filtering information through trusted network connections (Cann et al., 2011) and so helping to minimize a sense of information overload. Conversations across networks may identify topics for research or signpost researchers to funding opportunities or to new collaborators. The use of hashtags can help tracking conversations and content. Hashtags are words, acronyms or unspaced phrases preceded by the # symbol, used to tag or label posts, content and conversations in SoMe sites, which can then be found by searching for that particular hashtag. The emergence of Symplur (Symplur, 2014) as a register and archive of healthcare hashtags provides a large databank of Twitter conversations around healthcare across all specialities including psychiatry. SoMe as a source of big data can be integrated with other offline data sources and monitored to gain an insight into current trends, and to identify opportunities in research (Ovadia, 2009) or potential collaborators. SoMe has changed the flow of information and led to a democratization of information (Quinton, 2013). Researchers can review this data, and join online conversations and networks, making it possible to crowd-source research ideas and involve patient groups in the co-design and production of research (Henderson et al., 2013; Ho, 2014).

Development

As a research idea is explored, social citation tools such as Mendeley, Zotero, Colwiz and CiteULike can be used to support a literature review around an initial idea (Allen et al., 2013; Cann et al., 2011; Fausto et al., 2012; Gardois et al., 2012; Ovadia, 2013; Shema et al., 2012). Interest groups exist in all of these sites, again supporting connectiveness and networking. A search in Mendeley for groups focusing on 'mental health' revealed 83 groups (Mendeley, 2014).

Individuals can create a project group in any of these tools, whilst Colwiz also offers research teams project management tools with shared calendars and tasks that can support project development. Google Drive and Google Docs support collaborative writing, social commenting and development of surveys (e.g. Cann et al., 2011), whilst tools like Evernote with its shared notebooks provide a way to share web clippings and other information to support project work. There are endless tools that can be used to support the development of a project. Communication tools such as Skype and Google Hangouts are particularly helpful for connecting collaborators across institutions and geographical regions, helping to reduce both the costs and time needed for travel (Cann et al., 2011; Nicholas & Rowlands, 2011).

Implementation

Many SoMe tools in a PRE can also be used in the implementation phase of a project. Some researchers

may blog about their own work or post queries and problems to their PRN on Facebook, Academia.edu, etc., which can be solved by the collective wisdom of the network (Bartling & Friesike, 2014; Cann et al., 2011).These tools complement traditional approaches to research throughout the project lifecycle. SoMe have also emerged as a mechanism for support across research communities. An example is #PhDChat (Ford et al., 2014), a Twitter chat which has developed into an international community providing mutual support and advice for both full-time and part-time PhD researchers across multiple disciplines including education, the humanities and healthcare.

As previously highlighted, SoMe, as well as supporting the research process may be the focus of the actual research as either a source of big data or as a means to recruit and interact with research subjects. Where this is the case it plays a pivotal role in the implementation of the project and we explore this in further detail below as we consider SoMe as the focus of research.

Dissemination

As the research cycle reaches its conclusion with publication and dissemination of findings, SoMe can help break down the boundaries between research communities and the wider public (Fordis et al., 2011). Publication in mainstream peer-reviewed journals continues to have high currency and is essential for all researchers in terms of career progression. Whilst some researchers blog, there is still wariness of content published on blogs due to the lack of peer review; indeed, this is seen as a barrier to engaging with new forms of scholarly communication despite emerging views that the current form of peer review will become unsustainable (Procter et al., 2010). There are calls to move from filtering before publication to filtering post publication (Mandavilli, 2011; Smith, 2010). In the worlds of mathematics and physics, public discourse on a paper before publication is common and this debate is now seen on blogs (Mandavilli, 2011).

In medicine, post-publication discourse is occurring via Twitter on hashtags such as #FOAMed (Nickson, 2014), blogs (Shema et al., 2012) and open journal clubs running on Twitter and Facebook, including #BlueJC, which is supported by the *British Journal of Obstetrics and Gynaecology* (Leung et al., 2013). Platforms such as Academia.edu have plans to launch a post-publication peer review feature to serve as a filtering mechanism and help academics identify which research can be trusted (van Noorden, 2014). As SoMe tools are used to comment on and share, research altmetrics ('alternative metrics') provide a mechanism to measure the wider reach and social impact of scholarly work supplementing the traditional notions of citation impact and Hirsch number (Fausto et al., 2012; Kwok, 2013; Ovadia, 2013). Altmetrics serve to quantify the social activity around individual publications, and journals are beginning to display the social mentions of a paper including how many times a paper has been tweeted, saved to reference tools such as Mendeley and CiteULike, shared on Facebook, Google+, LinkedIn or blogged about. Social sharing options on publications make it easier to share research, and sharing articles via SoMe increases their dissemination (Allen et al., 2013). Social sharing leads to serendipitous discovery of academic work, which is now playing an important role alongside active searches of the literature (Dantonio et al., 2012). For work published in niche fields of research, a good paper may not have as good an altmetric as a 'middle of the road paper' in a mainstream research area (Kwok, 2013) and so some caution should be taken in interpreting these new metrics. Kwok does report, however, that there are signs in some quarters such as the UK's Research Excellence Framework of researchers being allowed to include altmetrics as evidence of the social impact of their research.

SoMe, and blogging in particular, can increase the accessibility of research from high impact journals. Psychiatry, neuroscience and psychology are well represented in scholarly blogs (Shema et al., 2012). Meanwhile, patient blogs are widely read and support the development of networks around them. However, they are less likely to refer to published research, given that research outputs are typically published behind paywalls, and are less well connected to blogs written by doctors (Gruzd et al., 2012a). Wider adoption of SoMe by researchers to communicate health information has the potential to impact on public opinion and to address misinformation, particularly in relation to public health issues (Foulkes, 2011). Blogging research can also help its discoverability, making it more likely to come up in Internet search engines; it may also lead to more accurate reporting in the media (Kumar, 2014). Furthermore, sharing of conference research presentations on Slideshare, or publishing podcasts and videos to YouTube can also help to better inform the public on health issues. Open online digital repositories such as Figshare (http://figshare.com) offer another option for researchers to publish their research data and outputs in a citeable and shareable way that supports the principles of open science. This open approach to sharing research outputs and engagement with the public can help the research come full circle and the resulting SoMe mediated dialogue may in turn lead to new research opportunities. It would also serve to raise the profile of work and perhaps has the potential to attract the attention of possible funders.

A key issue for researchers engaging in the use of SoMe is the potential for work in the digital domain to be valued and considered as a criterion for promotion or tenure. Dissemination and publishing academic discourse on social media platforms is not generally acknowledged within promotion criteria and is rarely rewarded (Czerniewicz, 2013). This lack of recognition sends a message to the academic community that this work is not recognized or of value and consequently can deter researchers from engaging with social media and reaping the wider benefits it may bring, such as new collaborative and research opportunities. The absence of reward is also lamented by those engaged with activities such as blogging as typified in a blog post by Skeptical Scalpel (2014) which highlights that blogs may be much more widely read than chapters in books that no one will buy. The value of discourse around blogs critically appraising research and the impact these may have on improving patient outcomes is unacknowledged and has no currency in academia. Digital scholarship supported by SoMe needs to be recognized as scholarly activity which is of equal value to traditional publishing and not just a sideshow. As Weller (2011) highlights, this can be a challenge as SoMe activity does not fit with current practices. Promotion criteria need to reviewed and reworked for the digital age. One approach might be to consider a portfolio approach including metrics, evidence of impact, digital outputs and research community endorsements (Weller, 2011). Until these issues are addressed and contributions are recognized and rewarded, many researchers will continue to question whether it is worth investing time engaging with SoMe.

Adams & Barndt's (1978) adapted model proved particularly useful to obtain a general overview of SoMe in research, the tools employed in the various stages and some practical and ethical issues (Table 1). However, as anticipated above, in the next section we will use a different approach to better report the complex status of SoMe throughout the research stages which came across during the preliminary analysis reported above.

Social media as data

Increasingly SoMe is becoming the subject of research itself, and there has been a proliferation of scholarship in this area across different fields and disciplines (van Osch & Coursaris, 2014). As outlined above, we identified two distinct areas in which research using SoMe as data can be considered based on Moreno et al. (2013), namely observational and interactive. Within the observational domain, open data on SoMe channels such as Twitter or YouTube may be the focus of the research (e.g. Bruns & Burgess, 2012; Giglietto et al., 2012; Golder & Macy,

Table 1. SoMe use and tools in a research lifecycle.

	Phase 1 Planning	Phase 2 Development and engagement	Phase 3 Implementation	Phase 4 Dissemination
Use	Identifying opportunities and topic; Networking with and finding collaborators; Reviewing literature initially literature review – using SoMe as a search tool; Defining research questions	Detailed literature review: managing citations/literature; Research methodology: qualitative – quantitative – mixed methods; Theory and framework for research; Project management; Collaboration with others	Recruit and retain subjects; Access to hard to reach if not invisible populations; SoMe as big data/data already posted and available, which allows: Observation of online behaviours in a 'naturalistic' fashion (field research); Collection of naturally occurring data generated by members of the public in real/near real time; Collection of user metrics; Sentiment analysis; Social network analysis; Data unaffected by observation (no researcher's bias)	New models of open publishing – sharing what has not worked as well as what has; Conferences; Publication; Altmetrics; Public engagement in research communities; Open digital repositories
Tools	Open source journals, Blogs, (self-published work, research); Research communities, e.g. through Linkedin, Researchgate; Twitter; Google+; Symplur	Research communities, e.g. through Linkedin, Researchgate, academia.edu; Collaboration, e.g. through Google+, G Docs, Blogs, Twitter, Mendeley, Colwiz, Zotero, CiteULike	Twitter, Facebook; Online discussion forums; Blogs; YouTube; Symplur	Publishing platforms, e.g. Blogs, Slideshare, Scribd, Flickr; Open data repositories, e.g. Figshare; Research communities, e.g. LinkedIn, Researchgate, academia.edu; Broadcasting, e.g. Twitter, Facebook
Issues	Researchers' digital literacy; Ethical issues involved in using open SoMe data	Dynamics involving trust, independence, intellectual property amongst researchers (Das et al., 2014)	Demographic detail often missing (age, gender, ethnicity) or fake accounts; Challenges in recruitment; Absence of contact with the population studied decreases bias but can create other problems, in particular those relating to informed consent and protection of the subject (McKee, 2013); Ethical issues re using open SoMe data and consent for follow-up studies; Perceptions and understanding of privacy; Boundaries between public and private are blurred in SoMe, raising issues around: Consent Public trust Storage of data Ownership of data	Perceived trustworthiness of content by public, fellow researchers and academics (Gruzd et al., 2012a; O'Connor, 2013; Procter et al., 2010); Altmetrics interpretation (Kwok, 2013)

2013). Research in the interactive domain may involve recruiting subjects via SoMe channels such as Facebook (e.g. Balfe et al., 2012; Bull et al., 2011, 2013; Child et al., 2014; Kapp et al., 2013; Leonard et al., 2014) or be implemented through SoMe channels to answer specific questions (e.g. Quinton, 2013), with subjects being recruited and asked to use SoMe to record reflections and experiences on blogs or other platforms (e.g. Harricharan & Bhopal, 2014). In this way new data is produced by participants' engagement through SoMe.

We adapted and used Moreno et al.'s categorization of research approaches to discuss our findings in the following way.

1. Observational research: which does not require researchers to interact with human subjects to access and collect the data where SoMe is open research data.
2. Interactive research: when researchers contact participant(s) to either ask them to create content online or ask permission to view already existing content that is not publicly available. Here SoMe serves to recruit and retain participants and is used to create new data.

We supplement this discussion with some ethical considerations that emerged from the literature.

Social media in the observational domain

Individuals are increasingly sharing their lives on public SoMe spaces, which can be viewed as open laboratories (Giglietto et al., 2012) or public parks (Swirsky et al., 2014). Twitter is particularly public, and individual tweets can be read without owning a Twitter account. Tweets are referred to in news stories and provide a social, real time commentary around local, national and international news as well as natural disasters and unfolding flu outbreaks (Bruns & Burgess, 2012). By virtue of application programming interfaces (APIs – pieces of programming that allow addition and integration of features into various applications), tweets around search terms, or more typically, individual hashtags, which serve to support conversations around discreet topics, can be harvested and exported. Various tools can be used to export Twitter data: there are paid-for services such as Hashtracking, Keyhole or Tweetreach, and open-source tools such as Twitter Archiving Google Spreadsheet (TAGS) (Hawksey, 2013). It is different for Facebook, where individuals are more likely to have different privacy settings, so that conversations and postings amongst friendship groups (Giglietto et al., 2012) are often not so publicly visible. Public Facebook postings can, however, also be a rich source of open data as evidenced by

Moreno et al.'s (2013) study of college students disclosing symptoms of depression.

Twitter's privacy policy highlights the public nature of tweets stating, 'What you say on Twitter may be viewed all around the world instantly' (Twitter, 2014a). The policy draws users' attention to the fact that tweets are instantaneously delivered to search engines making clear that universities and public health agencies may analyse information shared via Twitter for trends and insights. Twitter recognizes that, with more than 500 million tweets being sent a day and the big data set this trend is generating, researchers may wish to explore it, particularly in relation to health, and is actively supporting the research community with its Data Grants programme (Twitter, 2014b). Whilst other SoMe sites do not mention that content posted may be the subject of research (Facebook, Tumblr, YouTube), they do highlight the public visibility and accessibility of posts, blogs, videos and comments, etc., and that these may be shared more widely. Users may have some degree of anonymity depending on their profile settings and the content posted, but cannot be guaranteed confidentiality with respect to any content. There are also issues of ownership, for example when posting a video on YouTube a user grants YouTube a worldwide, non-exclusive, royalty-free licence to use and reproduce their content. Facebook has different levels of privacy which may not be well understood by users and indeed Facebook users can be taken aback to discover that their profiles and postings are publicly viewable (Moreno et al., 2013).

It is against this backdrop of open big data that observational research of SoMe is undertaken. Twitter constantly provides real time data, news stories unfold and communities and networks form around common interests defined by hashtags (Bruns & Burgess, 2012). This bank of ever-growing big data is also seemingly opening up access to traditionally 'difficult to reach' groups, sometimes perceived as 'invisible populations' (Edwards et al., 2013). Near real-time analysis of Twitter data and computational methods can be used to support anticipation modelling, predict social problems, environmental hazards, health epidemics and identify new methods for disseminating health information (e.g. Edwards et al., 2013; Heaivilin et al., 2011). YouTube, with its public profiles and video uploads, has similarly become a focus for research in mental health (Naslund et al., 2014). Patients posting video narratives provide an insight into coping mechanisms, and qualitative thematic analysis of comments can highlight the levels of naturally occurring, meaningful peer support amongst individuals with severe mental illness occurring on YouTube. A strength of this observational approach identified in various studies (e.g. Child et al., 2014; Edwards et al., 2013; Fordis et al., 2011;

Heaivilin et al., 2011; Moreno et al., 2011, 2013; Walker, 2014) is the ability to observe real-life data without any interference from the researcher(s).

There are, however, also limitations, for example insights into an individual's motivation to post or create and upload videos cannot be collected, and the impact of the postings on viewers and other commenters also cannot be assessed. A study of eating disorder blogs on Tumblr (Gies & Martino, 2014) additionally suggested another drawback of researching open blog posts in relation to sampling. As blogs are updated with new postings over time, the themes emerging from a thematic analysis of postings may vary if compared with another sample of blogs over a different period of time. Therefore, to triangulate and integrate findings, the authors recommend applying grounded theory to future research in this area to see if other themes and concepts emerge in blogs focusing on specific issues such as eating disorders. Naslund et al. (2014) and Gies & Martino (2014) highlight that they would have liked to have followed up and contacted some of the bloggers to administer questions to further support their findings. This is a theme which has emerged in other SoMe observational studies (e.g. Kaye et al., 2012; Mychasiuk & Benzies, 2012; Parsi & Elster, 2014; Taylor et al., 2014), and has also raised ethical concerns where researchers may feel an obligation to follow up for potential 'lifesaving' benefits, personal safety or legal reasons (e.g. Swirsky et al., 2014, Taylor et al., 2014).

Methodological considerations

Although SoMe platforms were not designed to be research tools (Swirsky et al., 2014) they have rapidly become the focus of research and developed into forums for online intervention studies (Koskan et al., 2014). There is a clear need to develop methodological frameworks and theoretical grounding for SoMe research (van Osch & Coursaris, 2014) and as more work is done in this field these will emerge over time. Research to date has adopted quantitative and qualitative approaches as well as mixed methods (van Osch & Coursaris, 2014). Computational methods (Giglietto et al., 2012) and ethnographical approaches are also being used to look closely at the social interactions and analyse the social meaning of data to gain understanding of illness (Naslund et al., 2014). Together with statistical methods supporting the textual analysis of comments from YouTube or tweets to show how words or phrases are connected and how often they occur, discourse analysis (Lomborg, 2012) and ethnography-focused research are helping to make sense of the community and the sentiment of discourse (e.g. King et al., 2013; Konijin et al., 2013). Grounded theory approaches also appear to

be particularly helpful in analysing large corpora of online text (e.g. Gruzd et al., 2012a, 2012b; Harricharan & Bhopal, 2014).

One of the challenges around analysing data from SoMe platforms is that they cannot be easily compared, as different platforms produce different datasets and have different models of openness and licensing (Giglietto et al., 2012). This in turn suggests that different approaches need to be taken depending on the platform and the nature of the data being researched. The literature proposes metrics to support analysis of Twitter (Bruns & Stieglitz, 2013) and highlights other areas of analysis which could be undertaken on SoMe (e.g. Baker, 2013; Heaivilin et al., 2011; Hemsley et al., 2014). Bruns & Stieglitz (2013) proposed a set of metrics to support analysis of Twitter data which, if adopted, could help support the comparison of data across a range of studies and also lead to a greater scholarly exchange around research of big SoMe data. For example, researchers may wish to explore #depression on Twitter and compare conversations around this hashtag following significant media stories or during public health campaigns. A tweet provides information on the individual user including their Twitter name, the screen name of the user, a link to their profile and often their primary location, their profile picture/avatar, the date and time the tweet was posted, and – if they have enabled geolocation – the location from where the tweet was sent. This Twitter data can be used to measure activity around a hashtag or search term, the visibility of users, and a picture of activity over time. In addition, social network analysis (SNA) can provide an insight into the dynamics of the interaction and connections around a hashtag whilst sentiment analysis can give insight into mood of Twitter conversations, and manual content analysis allows for more thematic analysis of the tweets. Ford et al.'s (2014) analysis of the #PhDchat on Twitter demonstrates how these metrics can be applied to reveal the dynamics of a SoMe-mediated community and the themes typically discussed.

Further notes of caution are emerging in relation to the representation of differing groups and the authenticity or provenance of accounts or comments. This is particularly so in relation to Twitter, where researchers have highlighted that Twitter users are not necessarily representative of the wider population (Bruns & Burgess, 2012; Bruns & Stieglitz, 2013; Giglietto et al., 2012; Heaivilin et al., 2011; King et al., 2013; Ovadia, 2009); but the same issue has also been highlighted in relation to other SoMe (e.g. Swirsky et al., 2014; Wang et al., 2014). Individuals may also not be who they appear to be, due to lack or unreliability of demographic information such as gender, age, ethnicity or social class on sites such as Twitter, YouTube and

Tumblr. Additionally, with the use of pseudonyms and individuals adopting multiple personas, caution is advised against drawing conclusions applicable to the wider population (Quinton, 2013). Edwards et al. (2013) described SoMe data as 'surrogate data', which can only augment traditional data, and caution against using SoMe in isolation, due to their limitations. With an increasingly networked society and new social structures forming, Edwards et al. (2013) also question whether online networks exhibit the same openness and behaviour as offline networks. There are complex issues around identity which can come into play, with postings on SoMe not necessarily truly reflecting the opinions of the individual/s concerned (Boyd, 2014).

Ethical considerations

Researching open, publicly accessible data can have some benefits, such as the absence of the researcher's bias (McKee, 2013), but raises some ethical issues. Moreno et al. (2013) highlight the need to clearly define whether the research project is or is not about human subjects. When the information to be analysed is public and it does not require interaction with a human subject in order to access it, then the research is purely observational. This would be the case for studies in which only public data were evaluated to make collective observations (Moreno et al., 2013). For example Heaivilin et al. (2011) used Twitter to evaluate whether information relating to dental pain is broadcast on this media and assessed the content of the information being communicated; King et al. (2013) analysed the role of Twitter in the debate and sharing of information in a specific area of health policy; Gruzd et al. (2012a) evaluated blog posts to determine how often biomedical literature is referenced in blogs on diabetes and how these blogs interconnect with others in the health blogosphere. While these studies can be defined as observational, ethical and privacy issues are still pertinent. Researchers undertaking an observational study on SoMe should be aware of some elements regarding this fundamental debate, as highlighted in various studies (e.g. Eastham, 2011; McKee, 2013; Moreno et al., 2013), such as users' privacy settings, the website/service statements on privacy and use (as described above) and some legal considerations (Moreno et al., 2013).

Users' privacy settings are the most immediate element to be considered when undertaking observational research. In general, all SoMe services allow some degree of privacy to be set at users' discretion. Twitter allows users to set their tweets private, so that only specific people – the ones that have been 'accepted' as 'followers' – can read them. Otherwise tweets are visible to anyone on the Internet. Face-

book has a more complicated array of privacy settings, allowing users' profile information and posts' visibility to be regulated on various degrees of 'openness', from 'open to the public' (however, only visible to other Facebook users) to 'closed', only visible to 'friends', groups of friends or even only to themselves. Blog and video platforms have different visibility options which can be personalized to bloggers' preferences. A blog, and its content, can be made visible or hidden to search engines, it can be made private, a post or the whole blog only accessible to chosen users. Additional options include restricting comments to posts, in this way opening for discussion or being a read-only blog.

While such settings are rather straight forward for users, privacy, far from being a fixed or defined element of online content, is a dynamic entity that can change over time within the same user's content and connections. The dichotomy between public and private has been described as a discursive process where privacy is continuously negotiated within contexts and amongst users (Gal, 2002, cited in Eastham, 2011). For this reason, even when online content is public, researchers need to assess the private/public nature in order to develop inclusion or exclusion criteria (Eastham, 2011). Eastham (2011), talking about blogs in particular, advises researchers to look for 'clues regarding a blogger's intended public or private writing' (p. 355). Such cues are provided by the choices bloggers make in setting up their blogs, for example the use of pseudonyms to preserve anonymity, and the blog privacy settings. A blog that is available to search engines, has open content, allows readers to comment, and provides a really simple syndication feed (RSS), suggests that the author's intention is that the blog is considered public (Eastham, 2011). When any of these cases do not apply, the blogger's intentions on the publicity of his/her content is less evident and needs to be carefully evaluated.

Another important point highlighted by Eastham (2011) is the risk of identification of the blog author/s through the quotations used by the researcher in a publication. The author therefore suggests 'paraphrasing rather than using direct quotations' (p. 358), other than – obviously – anonymizing the quotation. This can be applied to any public source, not only blog posts. If in doubt, researchers may ask for consent (Eastham, 2011), but in this case they would be leaving the area of a purely observational study, moving to that of an interactive study. Researchers may also decide to completely exclude the source or use Bruckman's (2002, cited in Eastham, 2011) higher level of disguise (changing names, changing pseudonyms, omitting proper names of cities, schools, or businesses that might identify the blog author).

As highlighted by Moreno et al. (2013), this kind of research can get exemption from IRB review. However, this does not include cases in which subjects can be identified either directly or indirectly through data reports, or when subjects' data are disclosed outside the published research, putting them at risk of criminal or civil liability or reputation damage.

Social media in the interactive domain

Alongside being a natural source of big data, SoMe also offer many opportunities to support online research methods (ORMs). Research can be designed and implemented through SoMe to answer specific research questions (Quinton, 2013), and may bring specific benefits around recruiting participants who are traditionally hard to reach (Quinton, 2013; O'Connor et al., 2014). In health-related research it can be difficult to recruit participants around sensitive topics and ensure anonymity. Walker (2014) suggests that recruitment via SoMe can address this issue, as well as help recruit patients who may have difficulty attending more traditional focus groups, though this may depend on the SoMe platform used (Bull et al., 2013).

Social media to recruit and retain participants

The value of SoMe in recruiting and retaining research participants has been highlighted in various studies on different domains (Balfe et al., 2012; Bull et al., 2011, 2013; Child et al., 2014; Das et al., 2014; Kapp et al., 2013; Leonard et al., 2014; Morris, 2013; Mychasiuk & Benzies, 2012). Within the literature analysed in this study, the most common tools used for recruitment and retention were Facebook (Balfe et al., 2012; Child et al., 2014; Kapp et al., 2013; Mychasiuk & Benzies, 2012) and Twitter (O'Connor et al., 2014) or both, in combination (Leonard et al., 2014; Morris, 2013).

In the medical research domain SoMe are being employed by 'participant-centred initiatives' (PCIs) to facilitate participants' engagement and to encourage interaction and dialogue with the researchers (Kaye et al., 2012). According to Kaye et al. (2012) this approach can improve participants' recruitment and retention while improving quality and public confidence in research. SoMe is also cost-effective (Balfe et al., 2012), bringing savings on travel costs and time travelling to different hospitals and clinics as well as on postage costs, where mailshots would be used to recruit patients. Furthermore SoMe can be used by existing participants to recruit further research subjects by directly contacting friends or acquaintances, hence supporting snowballing sampling methods (e.g. Balfe et al., 2012; Child et al., 2014; O'Connor et al., 2014). With the snow-

balling action of retweets one tweet has the scope to be amplified and reach thousands of potential participants (O'Connor et al., 2014).

To deploy the full potential of SoMe, researchers may want to adopt some expedients to nurture a climate of trust within the research settings. For example, whilst the subjects may themselves remain anonymous, Walker (2014) proposes that researchers may need to reveal something of their own identity to develop trust with the research group. This might be done through creating a profile with a photograph and biography (e.g. O'Connor et al., 2014). This issue of trust was also raised by Balfe et al. (2012), who private messaged Facebook users asking them to participate in their diabetes study. Contrary to other cases (e.g. Child et al., 2014), this approach did not prove to be a successful recruitment method. The authors surmised that Facebook users may have concerns about the legitimacy of such requests, perhaps perceiving them as scams. They recommend that other researchers think carefully about how they might increase the perceived legitimacy of their messages with links to the project research homepage, for example. In relation to the issue of low yield in actual participation, other scholars highlight the need to clarify the role of Facebook as a data collection tool for healthcare studies, in order to unveil its full potential (Kapp et al., 2013).

Just as with SoMe as big data in the observational domain, consideration must be given to ethical issues, and cautions also apply about the truly representative nature of participants that may be recruited. Morris (2013) highlighted that people with disabilities may disproportionately be living in poverty and not have access to the Internet. Balfe et al. (2012) identified that the participants they recruited via Facebook were largely middle class whilst the subjects they recruited through a local hospital were from more disadvantaged backgrounds. They concluded that researchers should not dismiss and abandon more traditional modes of recruitment – e.g. in clinics – which resonates with Edwards et al.'s (2013) view that SoMe should not be used alone but to augment traditional methods. Another limitation of using online environments in research is that researchers have low control over distractions, or participants may share research information with other participants, putting the scientific integrity at risk (Child et al., 2014; Lipset, 2014, p. 231).

Social media to create data

Following initial contact through SoMe – or traditional methods – for recruitment aims, researchers may ask participants to use SoMe to produce data. Depending on the research methodology, there can be a wide array of possibilities in which SoMe can play a role in the production of data. SoMe support the hosting and sharing of text, audio, image and video, which can be analysed qualitatively or quantitatively. SoMe support connections between users, so that they can access other's online profiles (e.g. 'friending', 'following', etc.) and eventually communicate through the various platforms.

Qualitative research may involve soliciting reflective online diaries or blog posts (e.g. Harricharan & Bhopal, 2014) or even simply requiring participants to create a Twitter account, which could then be evaluated looking either at the content of tweets (e.g. Hemsley et al., 2014) or at the network structure, obtaining a macro-view of the research area (Gruzd et al., 2012a). Some issues have been identified regarding this method. In particular, Harricharan & Bhopal (2014, p. 336) have noted that 'soliciting blogs from research participants means collecting social data unnaturally in this online environment.' A researcher asking research participants to perform an action online, such as posting content in the form of blog posts, comments, tweets, etc., may be forcing this behaviour in people that do not normally engage in these kinds of activities. However, the authors add that the participants' right to withdraw from the research at any time can help bring balance to the research setting (Harricharan & Bhopal, 2014).

Conclusions

There is no doubt that there is growing interest and engagement with social media in research. Using social media in the research lifecycle and developing a PRE can help save time and enhance collaborative working. Publishing via SoMe and open platforms provides new opportunities to enhance dissemination of research and increase the accessibility of valid and reliable information for patients. Moreover, some data and unsuccessful research outcomes that would not typically be accepted by a traditional journal can be shared via SoMe and be of substantial value to the wider research community. While researchers using these methods may become 'in contention' with traditional scholarly practice (Costa, 2013, cited in Greenhow & Gleason, 2014), many researchers are also clearly benefiting from developing research networks mediated by SoMe, which in turn we believe have the potential to nurture virtual communities of practice in research. We share Greenhow and Gleason's (2014) view that an in-depth reflective work may help stakeholders in evaluating ways to integrate such practices into academia, while agreeing on acceptable publishing outlets, including open access journals (p. 400). The one benefit that remains elusive for researchers is academic recognition and reward for those actively engaged with SoMe to disseminate research and impact on practice in

their field. There is a sense that this has become 'the elephant in the room' that needs to be addressed through open debate. Academia needs to review the rapidly evolving open digital publishing spaces and associated analytics and develop new approaches and criteria that can inform reward, promotion and tenure that are fit for purpose in the digital age.

SoMe has also opened up the new world of big open data providing new observational insights into the lives of patients with mental health issues in real-time, including their coping mechanisms and online support networks. This data may prove useful in the development of practice, health policy and service provision, and particularly so where it is considered alongside more traditional sources and approaches to data collection. It also affords new opportunities to engage with patients, involving them in the co-creation of research (Quinton, 2013) and to pursue more patient-centric initiatives in medical research (Kaye et al., 2012). Ethical issues need to be considered, and there is a clear need for an ongoing dialogue involving ethics committees, researchers and participants to bring potential problems to the fore and find ways to address and overcome these (Henderson et al., 2013).

The field of SoMe in research, although rapidly evolving, is still in its infancy and there is a lack of theoretical grounding (van Osch & Coursaris, 2014). Further work is needed to help develop theoretical frameworks to support the use of SoMe in observational research. One approach to help address this need would be to analyse SoMe data through a variety of different socio-cultural lenses to begin to understand what is at play. The outputs of such research could then help inform the construction of theoretical frameworks to support and guide future research. While SoMe are being tested and evaluated for research, we urge research practitioners to undertake a praxis-based approach to collaboratively shape new practices based on context-related evidence, thereby helping to bridge the gap between research and practice (Young et al., 2013).

Declaration of interest: The authors report no conflicts of interest. The authors alone are responsible for the content and writing of the paper.

References

Adams, J.R., & Barndt, S.E. (1978). Organizational life cycle implications for major projects. *Project Management Quarterly, 9,* 32–39.

Allen, H.G., Stanton, T.R., Di Pietro, F., & Moseley, G.L. (2013). Social media release increases dissemination of original articles in the clinical pain sciences. *PloS One, 8,* e68914.

Attwell, G. (2007). Personal learning environments – The future of elearning? *eLearning Papers, 2,* 1–8.

Archibald, M.M., & Clark, A.M. (2014). Twitter and nursing research: How diffusion of innovation theory can help uptake. *Journal of Advanced Nursing, 70,* e3–5.

Baker, S. (2013). Conceptualising the use of Facebook in ethnographic research: As tool, as data and as context. *Ethnography and Education, 8*, 131–145.

Balfe, M., Doyle, F., & Conroy, R. (2012). Using Facebook to recruit young adults for qualitative research projects: How difficult is it? *Computers, Informatics, Nursing, 30*, 511–515.

Bartling, S., & Friesike, S. (2014). Towards another scientific revolution. In S. Bartling, & S. Friesike, *Opening Science*. Berlin: Springer Open, pp.44, 1–12.

Boyd, D. (2014). *It's Complicated: The Social Lives of Networked Teens*. New Haven: Yale University Press.

Bruns, A., & Burgess, J. (2012). Researching news discussion on Twitter. *Journalism Studies, 13*, 801–814.

Bruns, A., & Stieglitz, S. (2013). Towards more systematic Twitter analysis: Metrics for tweeting activities. *International Journal of Social Research Methodology, 16*, 91–108.

Bull, S.S., Breslin, L.T., Wright, E.E., Black, S.R., Levine, D., & Santelli, J.S. (2011). Case study: An ethics case study of HIV prevention research on Facebook: The Just/Us study. *Journal of Pediatric Psychology, 36*, 1082–1092.

Bull, S.S., Levine, D., Schmiege, S., & Santelli, J. (2013). Recruitment and retention of youth for research using social media: Experiences from the Just/Us study. *Vulnerable Children and Youth Studies, 8*, 171–181. doi:10.1080/17450128.2012.748238

Cann, A., Dimitriou, K., & Hooley, T. (2011). *Social Media: A Guide for Researchers* (pp.1–46). London: Research Information Network.

Child, R., Mentes, J., & Phillips, L. (2014). Using Facebook and participant information clips to recruit emergency nurses for research. *Nurse Res, 21*, 2010–2015.

Czerniewicz, L. (2013). Power and politics in a changing scholarly communication landscape. . Paper 23. In *Proceedings of the IATUL Conferences* Purdue University, Purdue ePubs. Retrieved from http://docs.lib.purdue.edu/iatul/2013/papers/23

Dantonio, L., Makri, S., & Blandford, A. (2012). Coming across academic social media content serendipitously. In *Association for Information, Science and Technology 2012* Baltimore, Maryland.

Das, S., McCaffrey, P.G., Talkington, M.W.T., Andrews, N.A., Corlosquet, S., Ivinson, A.J., & Clark, T. (2014). Pain research forum: Application of scientific social media frameworks in neuroscience. *Frontiers in Neuroinformatics, 8*, 21.

Davis, F.D. (1989). Perceived usefulness, perceived ease of use, and user acceptance of information technology. *MIS Quarterly, 13*, 319–340.

Eastham, L.A. (2011). Research using blogs for data: Public documents or private musings? *Research in Nursing and Health, 34*, 353–361.

Edwards, A., Housley, W., Williams, M., Sloan, L., & Williams, M. (2013). Digital social research, social media and the sociological imagination: Surrogacy, augmentation and re-orientation. *International Journal of Social Research Methodology, 16*, 245–260.

Facebook. (2014). Facebook's Privacy Policy. Retrieved 27 October 2014 from https://www.facebook.com/note.php?note_id=%20322194465300

Fausto, S., Machado, F.A, Bento, L.F.J., Iamarino, A., Nahas, T.R., & Munger, D.S. (2012). Research blogging: Indexing and registering the change in science 2.0. *PloS One, 7*, e50109.

Ford, K.C., Veletsianos, G., & Resta, P. (2014). The structure and characteristics of #PhDChat, an emergent online social network. *Journal of Interactive Media in Education, 8*. doi.org/10.5334/2014-08.

Fordis, M., Street, R.L., Volk, R.J., & Smith, Q. (2011). The prospects for Web 2.0 technologies for engagement, communication, and dissemination in the era of patient-centered outcomes research: Selected articles developed from the Eisenberg Conference Series 2010 Meeting. *Journal of Health Communication, 16*(Suppl.1), 3–9.

Foulkes, M. (2011). Social contexts, social media, and human subjects research. *American Journal of Bioethics, 11*, 35–6

Gardois, P., Colombi, N., Grillo, G., & Villanacci, M.C. (2012). Implementation of Web 2.0 services in academic, medical and research libraries: A scoping review. *Health Information and Libraries Journal, 29*, 90–109.

Gies, J., & Martino, S. (2014). Uncovering ED: A qualitative analysis of personal blogs managed by individuals with eating disorders. *Qualitative Report, 19*, 1–15.

Giglietto, F., Rossi, L., & Bennato, D. (2012). The open laboratory: Limits and possibilities of using Facebook, Twitter, and YouTube as a research data source. *Journal of Technology in Human Services, 30*, 145–159.

Golder, S.A, & Macy, M.W. (2013). Social media as a research environment. *Cyberpsychology, Behavior and Social Networking, 16*, 627–628.

Greenhow, C., & Gleason, B. (2014). Social scholarship: Reconsidering scholarly practices in the age of social media. *British Journal of Educational Technology, 45*, 392–402.

Grosseck, G., & Holotescu, C. (2011). Academic research in 140 characters or less. Paper presented at the 7th international scientific conference'eLearning and Software for Education' eLSE, Bucharest, April 28–29.

Gruzd, A., Black, F.A., Ngoc, T., Le, Y., & Amos, K. (2012a). Investigating biomedical research literature in the blogosphere: A case study of diabetes and glycated hemoglobin (HbA1c). *Journal of the Medical Library Association, 100* 34–42.

Gruzd, A., Staves, K., & Wilk, A. (2012b). Connected scholars: Examining the role of social media in research practices of faculty using the UTAUT model. *Computers in Human Behavior, 28*, 2340–2350.

Harricharan, M., & Bhopal, K. (2014). Using blogs in qualitative educational research: An exploration of method. *International Journal of Research and Method in Education, 37*, 324–343.

Hawksey, M. (2013, February 15). Twitter Archiving Google Spreadsheet TAGS v5 [Blog post]. Retrieved from https://mashe.hawksey.info/2013/02/twitter-archive-tagsv5/

Heaivilin, N., Gerbert, B., Page, J.E., & Gibbs, J.L. (2011). Public health surveillance of dental pain via Twitter. *Journal of Dental Research, 90*, 1047–1051.

Hemsley, B., Palmer, S., & Balandin, S. (2014). Tweet reach: A research protocol for using Twitter to increase information exchange in people with communication disabilities. *Developmental Neurorehabilitation, 17*, 84–89.

Henderson, M., Johnson, N.F., & Auld, G. (2013). Silences of ethical practice: Dilemmas for researchers using social media. *Educational Research and Evaluation, 19*, 546–560.

Ho, K. (2014). Harnessing the social web for health and wellness: Issues for research and knowledge translation. *Journal of Medical Internet Research, 16*, e34.

Kapp, J.M., Peters, C., & Oliver, D.P. (2013). Research recruitment using Facebook advertising: Big potential, big challenges. *Journal of Cancer Education, 28*, 134–137.

Kaye, J., Curren, L., Anderson, N., Edwards, K., Fullerton, S.M., Kanellopoulou, N., .. Winter, S.F. (2012). Science and society: From patients to partners: Participant-centric initiatives in biomedical research. *Nature, 13*, 371–376.

King, D., Ramirez-Cano, D., Greaves, F., Vlaev, I., Beales, S., & Darzi, A. (2013). Twitter and the health reforms in the English National Health Service. *Health Policy, 110*, 291–297.

Konijn, E.A., Veldhuis, J., & Plaisier, X.S. (2013). YouTube as a research tool: Three approaches. *Cyberpsychology, Behavior and Social Networking, 16*, 695–701.

Koskan, A., Klasko, L., Davis, S.N., Gwede, C.K., Wells, K.J., Kumar, A., ... Meade, C.D. (2014). Use and taxonomy of social media in cancer-related research: A systematic review. *American Journal of Public Health, 104*, e20–37.

13

Kumar, M.J. (2014). Expanding the boundaries of your research using social media: Stand-up and be counted. *IETE Technical Review, 31*(4), 255–257.

Kwok, R. (2013). Research impact: Altmetrics make their mark. *Nature, 500,* 491–493. doi:10.1038/nj7463-491a

Leonard, A., Hutchesson, M., Patterson, A., Chalmers, K., & Collins, C. (2014). Recruitment and retention of young women into nutrition research studies: Practical considerations. *Trials, 15,* 23.

Leung, E.Y.L., Tirlapur, S.A., Siassakos, D., & Khan, K.S. (2013). #BlueJC: BJOG and Katherine Twining Network collaborate to facilitate post-publication peer review and enhance research literacy via a Twitter journal club. *BJOG : An International Journal of Obstetrics and Gynaecology, 120,* 657–660.

Lipset, C.H. (2014). Engage with research participants about social media. *Nature Medicine, 20,* 231. doi:10.1038/nm0314-231

Lomborg, S. (2012). Researching communicative practice: Web archiving in qualitative social media research. *Journal of Technology in Human Services, 30,* 219–231.

Mandavilli, A. (2011). Trial by Twitter. *Nature, 469,* 20.

McKee, R. (2013). Ethical issues in using social media for health and health care research. *Health Policy, 110,* 298–301.

Mendeley. (2014).Groups. Retrieved 6 November 2014 from http://www.mendeley.com/groups/search/?query = %22mental + health%22&page = 0

Moreno, M.A., Jelenchick, L.A., Egan, K.G., Cox, E., Young, H., Gannon, K.E., & Becker, T. (2011). Feeling bad on Facebook: Depression disclosures by college students on a social networking site. *Depression and Anxiety, 28,* 447–455. doi:10.1002/da.20805

Moreno, M.A., Grant, A., Kacvinsky, L., Moreno, P., & Fleming, M. (2012). Older adolescents' views regarding participation in Facebook research. *Journal of Adolescent Health, 51,* 439–444.

Moreno, M.A., Goniu, N., Moreno, P.S., & Diekema, D. (2013). Ethics of social media research: Common concerns and practical considerations. *Cyberpsychology, Behavior and Social Networking, 16,* 708–713.

Morris, R. (2013). 'Unjust, inhumane and highly inaccurate': The impact of changes to disability benefits and services – Social media as a tool in research and activism. *Disability and Society, 28,* 724–728.

Mychasiuk, R., & Benzies, K. (2012). Facebook: An effective tool for participant retention in longitudinal research. *Child: Care, Health and Development, 38,* 753–756.

Naslund, J.A., Grande, S.W., Aschbrenner, K.A., & Elwyn, G. (2014). Naturally occurring peer support through social media: The experiences of individuals with severe mental illness using YouTube. *PloS One, 9,* e110171. doi:10.1371/journal.pone.0110171

Nicholas, P.D., & Rowlands, I. (2011). Social media use in the research workflow. *Information Services and Use, 31,* 61–83.

Nickson, C. (2014, February 6). FOAM [Blog post] Retrieved 6 November 2014 from http://lifeinthefastlane.com/foam/

O'Connor, A., Jackson, L., Goldsmith, L., & Skirton, H. (2014). Can I get a retweet please? Health research recruitment and the Twittersphere. *Journal of Advanced Nursing, 70*(3), 599–609.

O'Connor, D. (2013). The apomediated world: Regulating research when social media has changed research. *Journal of Law, Medicine and Ethics, 41,* 470–483.

Ovadia, S. (2009). Exploring the potential of Twitter as a research tool. *Behavioral and Social Sciences Librarian, 28,* 202–205.

Ovadia, S. (2013). When social media meets scholarly publishing. *Behavioral and Social Sciences Librarian, 32,* 194–198.

Parsi, K., & Elster, N. (2014). Conducting research on social media – Is Facebook like the public square? *American Journal of Bioethics, 14,* 63–65.

Procter, R., Williams, R., & Stewart, J. (2010). If you build it, will they come? How researchers perceive and use Web 2.0. *Philosophical Transactions of the Royal Society A, 368,* 4039–4056.

Quinton, S. (2013). The digital era requires new knowledge to develop relevant CRM strategy: A cry for adopting social media research methods to elicit this new knowledge. *Journal of Strategic Marketing, 21,* 402–412.

Rowlands, I., Nicholas, D., Russell, B., Canty, N. & Watkinson, A. (2011). Social media in the research workflow. *Learned Publishing, 24,* 183–195.

Shema, H., Bar-Ilan, J., & Thelwall, M. (2012). Research blogs and the discussion of scholarly information. *PloS One, 7,* e35869.

Smith, R. (2010). Classical peer review: An empty gun. *Breast Cancer Research, 12,* S13.

Skeptical Scalpel. (2014, October 4) Should social media accomplishments be recognized by academia? [Blog post]. Retrieved 8 January 2015 from http://skepticalscalpel.blog spot.co.uk/2014/10/should-social-media-accomplishments-be.html

Swirsky, E.S., Hoop, J.G., & Labott, S. (2014). Using social media in research: New ethics for a new meme? *American Journal of Bioethics, 14,* 60–61.

Symplur. (2014). Why the Healthcare Hashtag Project? Retrieved 26 October 2014 from http://www.symplur.com/healthcare-hashtags/

Taylor, H.A., Kuwana, E., & Wilfond, B.S. (2014). Ethical implications of social media in health care research. *American Journal of Bioethics, 14,* 58–59.

Tumblr. (2014). Privacy policy. Retrieved 27 October 2014 from https://www.tumblr.com/policy/en/privacy

Twitter. (2014b). Twitter engineering blog – Introducing T witter data grants 05/02/2014. Retrieved 27 October 2014 from https://blog.twitter.com/2014/introducing-twitter-data-grants.

Twitter. (2014a). Privacy policy. Retrieved 27 October 2014 from https://twitter.com/privacy

Van Noorden, R. (2014). Scientists and the social network. *Nature, 512,* 126–129.

van Osch, W., & Coursaris, C.K. (2014). Social media research: An assessment of the domain's productivity and intellectual evolution. *Communication Monographs, 81,* 285–309.

Walker, D. (2014). The Internet as a medium for health services research. Part 2. *Nurse Researcher, 20,* 33–37.

Wang, C., Yang, J., Zhu, H., & Yu, L. (2014). Research on foreign tourists' satisfaction with the 2010 Shanghai World Expo: Based on the blogs at a travel website. *Journal of Convention and Event Tourism, 15,* 114–134.

Weller, M. (2011). *The Digital Scholar: How Technology is Transforming Scholarly Practice.* London: Bloomsbury.

Young, P.J., Nickson, C.P., & Gantner, D. (2013). Can social media bridge the gap between research and practice? *Critical Care and Resuscitation, 15,* 257–259.

YouTube (2014). Terms and conditions. Retrieved 27 October 2014 from https://www.youtube.com/static?template = terms

Ethical issues when using social media for health outside professional relationships

MATTHEW DECAMP

Berman Institute of Bioethics, Division of General Internal Medicine, Johns Hopkins University, Baltimore, Maryland, USA

Abstract

Social media have the potential to revolutionize health and healthcare, but fulfilling this potential requires attention to the ethical issues social media may raise. This article reviews the major ethical issues arising when social media are used for research, public health, mobile health applications, and global health. It focuses on social media use outside fiduciary relationships between healthcare professionals and patients. Emphasis is given to the potential of social media in these contexts, the ethical issues relatively unique to each, and where possible how existing ethical principles and frameworks could help navigate these issues. In some cases social media create the circumstance for particular ethical issues but also facilitate managing them, such as in informed consent for research. In other cases, disagreement exists about whether social media – despite their potential – should be used for certain purposes, such as in public health surveillance (where confidentiality represents a significant ethical concern). In still others, ethical uncertainty exists about how social media will affect ethical issues, such as inequality in global health. As social media technologies continue to develop, identifying and managing the ethical issues they raise will be critical to their success in improving health while preserving fundamental ethical values.

Introduction

With evidence consistently demonstrating increasing use of social media for health-related purposes (e.g. Fox, 2011), social media appear poised to truly revolutionize health and healthcare (Mayo Clinic Center for Social Media, 2012). Characterized by a collaborative, participatory, and open approach to information sharing and knowledge generation (Eysenbach, 2008), paradigmatic examples of social media – such as Facebook, Twitter, and others – are being used for a range of purposes related to health (Grajales et al., 2014; Moorhead et al., 2013). These uses include provision of medical care, public health, research, and medical education, among others.

Such rapid technological change can create new ethical issues or cause older issues to manifest in unique ways. It is unsurprising that social media by virtue of their collaborative, participatory and open nature have created worries about privacy and confidentiality, appropriate expertise online, and issues related to information sharing or appropriate personal/professional boundaries. Whether or not these worries are entirely new or threaten fundamental ethical values, addressing them is critical to ensuring social media are developed and used for health in ways that preserve these values.

This article reviews ethical issues in the use of social media for health, focusing on those occurring outside the context of professionalism. Although the distinction between ethics and professionalism is indistinct at best, for the purposes of this article, attention is given to issues arising outside the fiduciary relationships that form the basis of the special roles and responsibilities between healthcare professionals and their patients. As such, ethical issues related to social media and professional boundaries, telemedicine, electronic health records, and other healthcare applications within these relationships will not be directly covered. Indeed, some believe it is the very nature of social media technologies to function outside – or even question – traditional hierarchical professional relationships (Eysenbach, 2008; O'Connor, 2013).

This article instead emphasizes ethical issues in four different areas: research ethics, public health, mobile health applications, and global health. It describes existing evidence of social media's potential to impact health positively in these areas, notes examples where ethical concerns have been raised, and highlights the most salient ethical issues involved. A narrative approach is employed because of the relative nascence of social media in health, the topic's breadth, and its subject matter (ethics). To illustrate, the US National Library of Medicine's PubMed database includes the subject headings 'Ethics, research' (introduced in 2003) and 'Social media' (introduced in 2012). A combined search of these two headings yields three articles. Therefore, searches using combined keywords – 'social media', 'social networking', 'mHealth', 'ethics', and 'bioethics' for example – were used to generate a list of articles. These titles and abstracts were reviewed, with applicable articles reviewed in full and additional articles identified from works cited therein. Articles cited are meant to be representative; they are not intended as an exhaustive list or systematic review of the ethics literature.

Research ethics

Social media technologies have great potential to change the way health research is designed, conducted, and disseminated. Already, social media have been used in a number of research projects. Some use social media to help conduct traditional research projects, such as by facilitating health data collection within a social network (Weitzman et al., 2011). Others have used social media to fill specific research gaps, for example by recruiting research participants and conducting research within difficult to reach populations or about sensitive topics (such as adolescent substance abuse; see Ramo & Prochaska, 2012). Still others use social media as part of the research itself; for example, a recent study examining how Facebook users' emotions could be unknowingly manipulated has received considerable attention, as much for the ethical issues involved as for its findings of 'emotional contagion' (Kramer et al., 2014).

A novel and exciting part of social media in health research relates to participant-led research (Vayena & Tasioulas, 2013), defined broadly as research that is initiated and/or designed by the research participants themselves. In a notable example, individuals on PatientsLikeMe.com organized and conducted an investigation of lithium in amyotrophic lateral sclerosis (ALS) then published their results (Wicks et al., 2011). In another, social media were effectively used to organize a study of a rare condition, spontaneous coronary artery dissection (SCAD), helping facilitate a research investigation that might otherwise have languished (Tweet et al., 2011).

At the same time, ethical concerns have been raised about particular uses of social media. Controversy over the Facebook study of emotional contagion (Kramer et al., 2014) highlighted several ethical issues that arise when social media are used in research, including appropriate informed consent, the role of deception, and what counts as research requiring ethical oversight altogether. In the USA, the Secre-

tary's Advisory Committee on Human Research Protections (SACHRP) has attempted to apply and interpret fundamental research ethics principles of respect for persons, beneficence, and justice to the online setting (Secretary's Advisory Committee on Human Research Protections, 2013). Although uncertainty exists about how such research should be regulated (Kahn et al., 2014), researchers, research ethics committee members, and others can still consider a number of basic issues when health research involves social media (Moreno et al., 2013).

Design

As with the design and conduct of human subject research generally, a scientifically valid research design is prerequisite to the ethical conduct of social media research (Council for International Organizations of Medical Sciences, 2002). Otherwise, research participants may be subject to risks to no good purpose. In the social media setting, certain methodological issues could require special attention. These include biases related to self-selection of those who participate via social media, social desirability in the reporting of health states and information (e.g. under-reporting of substance abuse), and use of self-reported phenotypic data that would, in other contexts, be observed and collected by a third party (Janssens & Kraft, 2012).

Participant-led research (PLR) may present unique challenges to appropriate ethics oversight (Vayena & Tasioulas, 2013). In the research examining lithium and ALS, for example, the research team sought research ethics committee approval, perhaps partly because publication in the medical literature typically requires this. However, because ethical oversight relying upon research ethics committees ('institutional review boards' in the USA) is frequently attached to only certain institutional or regulation-defined entities – and because not all PLR will be published – formalized ethics review might neither occur nor be strictly required from a regulatory or legal perspective. Nevertheless, from the standpoint of ethics, to the extent that ethics review takes seriously the risks of harm to participants, review may be morally required. As a result, some have proposed novel methods of reviewing research before it proceeds past the design stage. Examples include crowd sourcing ethics review (i.e., having PLR protocols reviewed by online communities or on online forums, rather than by traditional in-person ethics committees) or the creation of citizen ethicists (i.e., members of the general public who volunteer to review PLR protocols) (Vayena & Tasioulas, 2013). Such novel methods have yet to be implemented, but might fill this regulatory gap and deserve further exploration.

Conduct

The conduct of research, while complex, involves several discrete steps, each of which is significant from an ethics standpoint. Each deserves attention in the setting of social media.

Recruitment

Individuals frequently learn about research via the recruitment process, and using social media as a tool for recruitment shows promise for improving recruitment and participation in health research (Allison, 2009; Blue Chip Patient Recruitment, 2011). Two fundamental aspects of ethics in recruitment involve ensuring that there is no untoward pressure for individuals to join a study and ensuring that subject selection is fair or equitable (i.e. that certain groups are not inappropriately recruited over others). In offline research, this could require conducting recruitment in an appropriate environment (e.g. by not recruiting in certain waiting room settings, such as at a substance abuse clinic) and ensuring that subject recruitment is not biased (e.g. in terms of gender, race, ethnicity, or socio-economic status, among others).

Recruitment via social media and social networks may present unique challenges for researchers. First, unlike the posting of recruitment flyers in a hallway or waiting room – where the research team has relative control over the message and where it is posted – both the brevity and potential viral spread of social media messages could complicate the recruitment environment. In terms of brevity, social media messages (such as 'tweets' of 140 characters on Twitter) are characteristically short. If research recruitment only includes such limited information, this could restrict the amount of information a potential research participant receives about a study. On the other hand, done well, social media recruitment could take advantage these technologies' capabilities to link to more detailed research study information and provide that information in dynamic, graphic and user-friendly forms when compared to traditional flyers.

In terms of viral message spread, researchers ought not be held responsible, in all cases, for where recruitment ads travel; however, they should realize that social media data analytics that promise to target specific geographic, racial, age, and other individual characteristics do so imperfectly, and that messages travel easily beyond their intended audience. Unlike an individual who passes by a potentially irrelevant research flyer, a misdirected social media recruitment ad about depression, substance abuse, or another sensitive topic appearing in an individual's social network could cause psychological or social distress in ways that traditional recruitment might not. In addition, although an individual can usually respond to a flyer confidentially (e.g. by writing down a telephone number from it), when he or she clicks the recruitment flyer online, this action may be recorded by the social media site – thereby affecting the individual's future social media content. Researchers should carefully consider these factors before recruiting for studies involving sensitive subject matters or using targeted ads.

Second, researchers should understand that recruitment within a social network may occur within a context where certain forms of social pressure to participate might exist (e.g. among Facebook friends). Although such recruitment may aid research involving rare diseases, when small or relatively tight-knit communities are involved, individuals may feel pressure to join a study occurring within their social network or may experience ostracism if they do not participate. To help avoid this disruption, researchers should engage with the social network community (e.g. by contacting site participants or moderators) prior to commencing recruitment in order to understand whether such pressures might exist.

Third, in terms of fairness or equity in recruitment, researchers should consider how the so-called digital divide (i.e. inequality in access to social media technologies) affects 'who' receives social media content, as well as how this divide is changing. Evidence suggests that this divide occurs more along age lines than it does race, gender, or traditional socio-economic factors (Duggan & Brenner, 2013). As research moves online, the implication is that fair and unbiased recruitment should be sensitive to the potential for age disparities in recruitment, perhaps more so than the more traditionally defined categories.

Consent

After individuals are recruited to participate in a study, they next consider whether to consent to join. Ethically, protecting individuals' autonomy requires obtaining valid informed consent. This is a key challenge for research in the social media setting (Vayena et al., 2012). Ethical challenges for informed consent in social media research include identity verification, ensuring participant understanding, and documenting the consent (Secretary's Advisory Committee on Human Research Protections, 2013).

There is general agreement that standards for identity verification, understanding, and documentation should vary depending on the research context (especially risk). For example, in research involving minimal or low risk, identity verification software might be sufficient to verify participant identity, and no test of understanding may be necessary. For research involving more risk, additional efforts including live chatting or messaging to answer participant questions, online tests of comprehension that must be passed to enrol in a study, or even the transmission of identity and/or standard consent documents could be required. By its nature, research involving minors presents a unique challenge and could require additional assurances regarding identity, parental consent, and understanding (Secretary's Advisory Committee on Human Research Protections, 2013). These additional assurances are sometimes legally required. For example, in the USA, the Children's Online Privacy Protection Act, or COPPA, (enacted in 1998 and made effective in 2000), requires parental consent before collecting, using, or disclosing information from individuals under the age of 13. However, for minors older than 13, the absence of such legal obligations underscores the need for attention to the ethical obligations regarding consent.

In some cases, innovative use of technology can help mitigate the challenges social media research presents for informed consent. For example, one challenge with informed consent via social media is that potential research subjects may not be engaged in a discussion with the researchers, because they 'read and click', rather than having conversations in person with researchers. A way to address this challenge could be to include times when researchers are online with potential subjects for secure chat sessions to answer questions about the study. At a more fundamental level, some have proposed rethinking the usual consent model into one that is 'collaborative and context-specific' consent, rather than a one-size fits all written document (Vayena et al., 2013). Under this model, for example, instead of simply moving written informed consent information online, the consent process would utilize innovative online technologies to present information in novel ways (e.g. graphically or dynamically over time). It could be 'collaborative', for example, by allowing potential subjects the opportunity to interact online with researchers or even other research participants at the time of their decision-making. It could be 'context-specific' by providing information to the subject based upon his or her personal characteristics, responses to questions posed about the research, or prior online activities. Tests of comprehension (e.g. about study details) could be included, requiring correct answers before proceeding to the next section. Such a tailored online consent process, while not yet widely available or used, could not only be a solution to the challenges created by social media research but also might be an improvement over standard written informed consent (Vayena et al., 2013).

Protecting privacy

Among risks attendant upon the design and conduct of social media research, protection of privacy risks is central (Thompson et al., 2011). Research involving social media has brought increased attention to the idea that information being 'online' is not equivalent to its being 'public'; in other words, online research is not equivalent to observation of public behaviour. On the other hand, online information is also not the same as paradigmatic examples of private information, such as medical records or personal diaries (Secretary's Advisory Committee on Human Research Protections, 2013). Protection of privacy in social media research must therefore be placed in context with how social media may be changing privacy norms themselves, as more individuals choose to share what was previously considered sensitive (O'Connor, 2013). In PLR, for example, participants voluntarily share a significant amount of health information. Significant uncertainty exists about what ethical protections, if any, are needed for such self-disclosures (including in the genetic context (Lee & Borgelt, 2014)).

Protecting privacy in the course of social media research thus requires researchers and others to identify when information should be considered 'private'. Keeping in mind the fundamental idea that 'online' is not equal to 'public', several criteria could assist researchers in this determination. First, it is incumbent upon researchers to understand the nature of the social media site where the research will be conducted, including its terms and conditions, and more especially what the expectations of site users are. Some health-related forums, for example, explicitly preclude research, and other forums may have their own norms and expectations. Second, when sites require a login or users are authorized to join by a site moderator in order to post content, this can reasonably interpreted as evidence of an expectation of privacy – even if the information is itself visible to the public on the Internet, as is true for some online patient forums. Third, when the site is organized around an express purpose – e.g. sharing of narrative stories – there might be a presumption that users share their stories with an expectation of privacy. Researchers would do well to consider carefully the nature of the social media environment where the research might occur and interact with its users or moderators in advance.

Community engagement

Health research increasingly emphasizes engaging patients in the research process. This is one focus, for example, of the US Patient Centered Outcomes Research Institute. The collaborative and participatory nature of social media create the potential for social media to help meet the fundamental ethical goals of community engagement in research, enhancing protection of research subjects, enhancing research benefits, improving the legitimacy of the research enterprise, and fostering shared responsibility over research (Dickert & Sugarman, 2005). Notably, social media have been used and evaluated to engage patients in studies proposing to conduct research in the emergency setting (Stephens et al., 2013).

However, social media at present may be best used to complement, not replace, more comprehensive engagement strategies that frequently include meetings and forums in person. A key question is whether social media effectively engage all potential research participants (e.g. the elderly, or non-English speakers), as well as whether or how to measure effective social media engagement (e.g. via web statistics or transcripts of web chats, among other possible means) (Chretien, 2013). Future research is needed to better understand how to use social media effectively for this purpose.

Public health

Although some ethical issues involved in using social media for public health overlap with those of research (Vayena et al., 2012), there are unique issues to consider in public health surveillance and interventions using social media. Social media have great potential to improve public health. For example, when traditional telephone lines were inoperative after the 2010 earthquake in Haiti, social media via cellular connections proved an invaluable part of disaster response (Merchant et al., 2011). Although evidence is limited (Kass-Hout & Alhinnawi, 2013; Velasco et al., 2014), surveillance of Internet and other search data may help predict influenza or other epidemics (Ginsberg et al., 2009; Corley et al., 2010). Social media may also play a role in public health interventions; for example, the USA's Centers for Disease Control and Prevention (2011) created a social media tool kit designed to help public health practitioners effectively spread health information.

Yet some applications of social media in public health may raise ethical concerns. Case reports of using Facebook to trace the contacts of an individual afflicted with a communicable disease caused some to wonder whether such uses – despite their effectiveness (Hunter et al., 2014) – represented a breach of confidentiality (Mandeville et al., 2014).

For public health uses of social media, major ethical issues that are well-recognized in public health include not only confidentiality, but also the protection of individuals' fundamental rights (such as liberty, which is most clearly involved in public health quarantine) and social justice for vulnerable or marginalized groups (Thomas et al., 2002). Ethics frameworks exist and can be used to help evaluate the ethics of social media when applied to public health (Kass, 2001). The following key questions from this framework can and should be applied to the public health setting.

1. What are the public health goals of the proposed social media programme?
2. How effective is the programme in achieving its goals?
3. What are the known or potential burdens of the programme?
4. Can the burdens be minimized, and are there alternative approaches?
5. Is the programme implemented fairly (i.e. with benefits and burdens fairly distributed among individuals and groups)?
6. How can the benefits and burdens of the programme be fairly balanced?

A hypothetical application of this framework to a proposed public health programme using social media demonstrates its utility in structuring important ethical values at stake. Imagine a programme that seeks to engage in both surveillance and intervention of a communicable disease, such as a sexually transmitted infection (STI). The programme proposes to actively monitor Twitter messages ('tweets') about the STI, analyse tweet content to estimate an individual's risk of possessing the STI, and then direct targeted messages to that individual to help reduce that risk.

The public health goals of this programme, which seem reasonable, are to improve public health STI control and reduce the risk of STI for the individual in question (question 1). Widespread implementation of this programme could only be justified if sufficient evidence exists regarding its effectiveness (question 2). As mentioned previously, however, known or potential burdens of the programme include privacy and confidentiality risks (question 3). Individuals targeted by these messages might feel as if their privacy had been breached by having their Twitter interactions monitored, or if inappropriately targeted, they might experience psychological distress. Here it becomes important to consider how to minimize these burdens and whether alternative approaches – even those not involving social media – might achieve the same goal without such burdens (question 4).

Next, the implementation of the programme must be evaluated according to fairness by taking into consideration whom it will target (question 5). Targeting an at-risk population (e.g. if a condition preferentially affects certain groups) is not necessarily unethical. However, in such cases it may be important to consult or engage with members of the group to help inform programme design, decision-making about how to make a final decision about the programme (question 6) and achieve buy-in. Applying an existing public health ethics framework (Kass, 2001) can therefore help identify the ethical issues involved in this social media intervention and even help effectively manage them.

Mobile health applications

Although social media and health has frequently focused on use by health professionals, broadly considered, attention is increasingly focusing on how social media – in particular, mobile health applications or 'apps' (sometimes known as 'mHealth') – can help patients improve their own health by providing them access to advice, allowing them to track their health conditions, and facilitating their sharing of health data among peers, friends, other patients with the same condition, or even health professionals (whether or not they have an existing professional relationship). For example, many apps exist for diabetes self-management, with some evidence of success (Goyal & Cafazzo, 2013). Mobile technologies may also be a way to engage hard-to-reach individuals or populations, such as adolescents, who not incidentally may be more likely to use mobile devices (Amicizia et al., 2013).

On the other hand, the evidence is not unequivocally positive for mobile applications. For example, a recent review of psychiatry and mental health related mobile applications revealed that many had hidden costs, lacked theoretical basis, and were of unproven effectiveness (Harrison & Goozee, 2014). A review in the area of cerebrovascular disease found that applications targeted towards healthcare professionals were more likely to be scientifically valid than those targeting patients (Dubey et al., 2014). Other disease-oriented applications such as in HIV care have had little uptake, with a need identified for greater collaboration between application developers and public health experts (Muessig et al., 2013); a systematic review of mobile applications for asthma found insufficient evidence to recommend their widespread use (Marcano Belisario et al., 2013).

These and similar findings have led some to advocate for greater regulation and governance of mobile health applications and related technologies (Charani et al., 2014). Ongoing efforts by the US Food and Drug Administration (FDA) (2013) and European Commission (2014) appear to be responsive to such calls.

Importantly, the debate over regulating social media and mobile applications has ethical components. Key terms of the debate are themselves ethical values: Protecting patients from harmful or ineffective applications, ensuring patients' data security, preserving patients' freedom of choice and empowerment, improving access to care, and appropriately stimulating innovation of new applications, and so on – as well as achieving a proper balance among them (Thompson & Brodsky, 2013) – are fundamentally about ethics. Hence the US FDA's (2013) guidance can be seen as striking a balance among these potentially competing ethical values. Its decision to regulate applications that interface with traditional medical devices (e.g. electrocardiographs and pacemakers) or transform a mobile device into a regulated one (e.g. by turning a mobile phone into an electrocardiography device) – but not a number of low risk devices (e.g. calorie counters or other devices based on standard reference information) – is an attempt to strike this balance. Whether the balance struck is the ideal one may be up for debate and requires further research.

An important ethical issue worth highlighting for mobile health applications is privacy. Users of mobile applications may be unaware that their health data are sometimes used by or sold to third parties. For example, when the US Federal Trade Commission reviewed 12 mobile health applications, it found that data were shared with 76 third parties (Federal Trade Commission, 2014). Such dissemination or selling of private information may carry benefits for users (e.g. through improved tailoring of the application or, in some cases, advertising), but it also carries risks of users' information being used without their knowledge or for purposes to which they might object.

A final ethical issue relating to consumer health applications involves the potential justice or fairness implications of mobile health. As previously noted, there is evidence that the digital divide (i.e. disparities in access to the Internet or other technologies) involves age more so than traditional characteristics such as race, ethnicity, or socio-economic status in developed countries such as the USA (Duggan & Brenner, 2013; Zickuhr et al., 2012). Nevertheless, health disparities persist within and between nations. As a matter of justice, a moral difference exists between allowing increased access to technology to improve the health of all ('a rising tide lifts all boats') and explicitly intending to ensure technology works to the preferential benefit of those experiencing health disparities ('special attention to those in need'). In other words, there may be an ethical rationale for ensuring new technologies benefit the so-called 'worst off' first, rather than waiting for technologies to 'trickle down' to these individuals. Whether existing regulations and activities around mobile health technologies will or should preferentially improve the health of socially marginalized and vulnerable groups is a critical but unanswered ethical question of justice (Pal, 2014).

Global health

Concern for equity in access and application of social media becomes arguably a more pressing issue when considering the persistent and drastic inequalities evident in global health. Access to digital technologies in developing countries has outpaced access to other basic goods and services, such as clean water, creating an opportunity for social media and mobile to leapfrog existing barriers to global health equity (Vital Wave Consulting, 2009; World Bank, 2012). Examples exists for the potential of social media and mobile health technologies to revolutionize medical education, the delivery of care, and public health surveillance activities worldwide (Betjeman et al., 2013; Hall et al., 2014). There have also been high profile, collaborative funding initiatives to simulate use of similar technologies globally (Gerber et al., 2010).

At the same time, the current evidence base for mobile applications and social media in global health, while promising, is limited to pilot-level programmes that need to be scaled and further tested (Hall et al., 2014). Global mental health in particular remains relatively unexplored (Farrington et al., 2014). In addition, some express appropriate skepticism that technology is unlikely to solve deeply entrenched disparities, particularly when other structural or systematic causes, such as poverty or social hierarchy, are involved (Barclay et al., 2014). Others have worried that interest in mobile health applications globally could be being driven more by donors than by the populations standing to benefit (Schuchman, 2014).

Although relevant in all contexts, of particular relevance to social media and global health is the ethical distinction between processes and outcomes. Understanding the distinction between fair processes (or procedural justice, emphasizing transparency ongoing evaluation and revision of decision-making; Daniels, 2000) and fair outcomes can help ensure the ethical use of social media for global health.

In light of past colonialism and ongoing disparities in economic and social power, ensuring that social media are implemented via fair processes is paramount. Fair processes will recognize that health technologies are not created paternalistically in developed countries and delivered to developing ones but instead seek to partner with local communities to develop technologies with them. Some have called this a 'people first' process-oriented approach (Barclay et al., 2014). The defining element of a 'people first' approach is engaging the individuals involved in, or affected by, decisions surrounding technology development and implementation. Engagement broadly construed seeks to ensure that the needs, values, and priorities of individuals are included in the decision-making process, thereby demonstrating respect for them as individuals and helping protect vulnerable groups (e.g. if they are explicitly included in the process). Engaging people in the process of technological development not only demonstrates the ethical value of respect; it also takes advantage of

their local knowledge in ways that may, in the end, help ensure technological uptake.

A critical and closely related process element important in the global context is ensuring that implementation is sensitive to cultural differences. Technology and its application may have different meanings or significance in different cultures, and in some cultures technological solutions (despite their effectiveness) might violate cultural norms and beliefs and thus be rightfully rejected. Those seeking to implement such technologies should be sensitive to these differences, lest they inadvertently violate cultural norms.

Outcomes – i.e. whether new social media technologies are actually used by people, or whether they improve health outcomes, reduce disease burden, and so on – are no less important, especially given the present absence of evidence demonstrating the effectiveness of social media applications globally. Not incidentally, an effective engagement process can help achieve effective outcomes by identifying in advance social factors that may be critical to programme success or by enhancing trust more generally. In terms of ensuring fair outcomes, however, key questions include whether the planned social media intervention is responsive to local needs, whether a plan exists for building capacity locally to solve the health problem, and the extent to which identified outcomes and effects (positive and negative) will be monitored and evaluated.

Joint emphasis on ethical processes and ethical outcomes can help ensure a 'people first' approach to implementing social media for global health. A people first approach will start by engaging a local community to help determine their health needs and priorities. It will then work to determine whether a mobile health or social media technology is even appropriate to meeting that need, and partner with them to develop that technology in ways that are culturally appropriate, feasible, and likely to be used by the community. Finally, it will continue to engage the community in evaluating the technology's real-world impact on the community's people and their health outcomes relevant to that need.

Conclusion

This article has reviewed ethical issues in the use of social media outside the traditional professional setting in research ethics, public health, mobile health applications, and global health. A few trends are worth noting. A common theme among all four contexts is the ethical importance of engagement – i.e. engaging social media sites and network in advance of a research project, engaging target groups before beginning a new public health intervention, engaging consumers in the creation of mobile health, and engaging global populations in the design of mobile health applications to meet their needs. Ethically, engagement demonstrates respect, helps ensure social media benefit users, and when combined with fair processes, could help improve social justice.

In general, the literature surrounding ethical issues in research and in public health is more extensive than the literature surrounding consumer health applications and global health. As a result, attention in research and public health has turned to exploring and evaluating – empirically – effective ways to manage these issues, such as in the development of novel forms of informed consent to protect autonomy in research. On the other hand, in consumer health and global health, a greater opportunity exists for additional conceptual work (e.g. regarding the appropriate balance of access and regulation for consumer health, or what counts as 'fairness' in terms of social media and the global digital divide).

Social media technologies are new and rapidly changing. However, the ethical values involved in their use for health are arguably not new, even if the distinct manifestation of the issues may be. In many cases existing ethical frameworks can be applied in this setting (e.g. in public health); in others, changes to ethical frameworks may be necessary as a result of how social media are shifting norms (e.g. in research ethics as a result of changing privacy norms). Importantly, just as social media may create the context for a particular ethical issue (e.g. the challenge of informed consent for research) they may also help facilitate the solution (e.g. by innovative means of social media-mediated informed consent processes).

The ethical issues identified in this review may transcend the somewhat artificial boundaries between research ethics, public health, mobile health applications, and global health. Together, however, the ethical principles, existing ethics frameworks, and ethical distinctions emphasized here can shape the way social media technologies develop. Because social media remain in their infancy, it will be important to continually reexamine the relationship between social media and ethics in healthcare, reiterating time-tested principles and frameworks where possible and updating them where necessary.

Declaration of interest: The author reports no conflict of interest. The author alone is responsible for the content and writing of the paper.

References

Allison, M. (2009). Can Web 2.0 reboot clinical trials? *Nature Biotechnology, 10,* 895–902.

Amicizia, D., Domnich, A., Gasparini, R., Bragazzi N.L., Lai, P.L., & Panatto, D. (2013). An overview of current and potential use of information and communication technologies for immunization promotion among adolescents. *Human Vaccines and Immunotherapeutics, 9*(12), 2634–2642.

Betjeman, T.J., Soghoian, S.E., & Foran, M.P. (2013). mHealth in sub-Saharan Africa. *International Journal of Telemedicine and Applications,* 482324.

Barclay, G., Sabina, A., & Graham, G. (2014). Population health and technology: Placing people first. *American Journal of Public Health, 104,* 2246–2247.

Blue Chip Patient Recruitment. (2011). *Engaging e-patients in clinical trials through social media.* Retrieved from http://bcpatientrecruitment.com/news/wp-content/uploads/2014/04/BlueChip_SocialMedia_5-2011.pdf

Centers for Disease Control and Prevention (US). (2011). *The Health Communicator's Social Media Toolkit.* Retrieved from http://www.cdc.gov/healthcommunication/toolstemplates/socialmediatoolkit_bm.pdf

Charani, E., Castro-Sanchez, E., Moore, L.S., & Holmes, A. (2014). Do smartphone applications in healthcare require a governance and legal framework? It depends on the application! *BMC Medicine, 12,* 29.

Chretien, K.C. (2013). Social media and community engagement in trials using exception from informed consent. *Circulation, 128*(3), 206–208.

Corley, C.D., Cook, D.J., Mikler, A.R., & Singh, K.P. (2010). Using web and social media for influenza surveillance. *Advances in Experimental Medicine and Biology, 680,* 559–564.

Council for International Organizations of Medical Sciences (CIOMS). (2002). *International Ethical Guidelines for Biomedical Research Involving Human Subjects.* Geneva: World Health Organization.

Daniels, N. (2000). Accountability for reasonableness. *British Medical Journal, 321,* 1300–1301.

Dickert, N., & Sugarman, J. (2005). Ethical goals of community consultation in research. *American Journal of Public Health, 95*(7), 1123–1127.

Dubey, D., Amritphale, A., Sawhney, A., Amritphale, N., Dubey, P., & Pandey, A. (2014). Smart phone applications as a source of information on stroke. *Journal of Stroke, 16*(2), 86–90.

Duggan, M., & Brenner, J. (2013). *The Demographics of Social Media Users – 2012.* Pew Internet & American Life Project. Retrieved from http://www.pewinternet.org/files/old-media//Files/Reports/2013/PIP_SocialMediaUsers.pdf

European Commission. (2014). *Green Paper on Mobile Health.* Retrieved from http://ec.europa.eu/information_society/newsroom/cf/dae/document.cfm?doc_id = 5147

Eysenbach, G. (2008). Medicine 2.0: Social networking, collaboration, participation, apomediation, and openness. *Journal of Medical Internet Research, 10*(3), e2.

Farrington, C., Aristidou, A., & Ruggeri, K. (2014). mHealth and global mental health: still waiting for the mH^2 wedding? *Globalization and Health, 10,* 17.

Federal Trade Commission. (2014). *Consumer generated and controlled health data.* Retrieved from http://www.ftc.gov/system/files/documents/public_events/195411/consumer-health-data-webcast-slides.pdf

Food and Drug Administration. (2013). *Mobile medical applications: Guidance for industry and Food and Drug Administration staff.* Retrieved from http://www.fda.gov/downloads/MedicalDevices/../UCM263366.pdf

Fox, S. (2011). *The social life of health information.* Pew Internet & American Life Project. Retrieved from http://www.pewinternet.org/files/old-media/Files/Reports/2011/PIP_Social_Life_of_Health_Info.pdf

Gerber, T., Olazabal, V., Brown, K., & Pablos-Mendez, A. (2010). An agenda for action on global e-health. *Health Affairs, 29*(2), 233–236.

Ginsberg, J., Mohebbi, M.H., Patel, R.S., Brammer, L., Smolinski, M.S., & Brilliant, L. (2009). Detecting influenza epidemics using search engine query data. *Nature, 457,* 1012–1014.

Goyal, S., & Cafazzo, J.A. (2013). Mobile phone health apps for diabetes management: Current evidence and future developments. *QJM: An International Journal of Medicine, 106,* 12, 1067–1069.

Grajales, F.J. III, Sheps, S., Ho, K., Novak-Lauscher, H., & Eysenbach, G. (2014). Social media: A review and tutorial of applications in medicine and health care. *Journal of Medical Internet Research, 16*(2), e13.

Hall, C.S., Fottrell, E., Wilkinson, S., & Byass, P. (2014). Assessing the impact of mHealth interventions in low-and middle-income countries – What has been shown to work? *Global Health Action, 7,* 25606.

Harrison, A.M., & Goozee, R. (2014). Psych-related iPhone apps. *Journal of Mental Health, 23,* 48–50.

Hunter, P., Oyervides, O., Grande, K.M., Prater, D., Vann, V., Reitl, I., & Biedrzycki, P.A. (2014). Facebook-augmented partner notification in a cluster of syphilis cases in Milwaukee. *Public Health Reports, 129*(Suppl.), 43–49.

Janssens, A.C., & Kraft, P. (2012). Research conducted using data obtained through online communities: Ethical implications of methodological limitations. *PLoS Medicine, 9,* e1001328.

Kahn, J.P., Vayena, E., & Mastroianni, A.C. (2014). Learning as we go: Lessons from the publication of Facebook's social computing research. *Proceedings of the National Academy of Sciences of the United States of America, 111*(38), 13677–13679.

Kass, N.E. (2001). An ethics framework for public health. *American Journal of Public Health, 91*(11), 1776–1782.

Kass-Hout, T.A., & Alhinnawi, H. (2013). Social media in public health. *British Medical Bulletin, 108,* 5–24.

Kramer, A.D.I., Guillory, J.E., & Hancock, J.T. (2014). Experimental evidence of massive-scale emotional contagion through social networks. *Proceedings of the National Academy of Sciences of the United States of America, 111*(24), 8788–8790.

Lee, S.S.-J., & Borgelt, E. (2014). Protecting posted genes: Social networking and the limits of GINA. *American Journal of Bioethics, 14*(11), 32–44.

Mandeville, K.L., Harris, M., Thomas, H.L., Chow, Y., & Seng, C. (2014). Using social networking sites for communicable disease control: Innovative contact tracing or breach of confidentiality? *Public Health Ethics, 7,* 47–50.

Marcano Belisario, J.S., Huckvale, K., Greenfield, G., Car, J., & Gunn, L.H. (2013). Smartphone and tablet self-management apps for asthma. *Cochrane Database of Systematic Reviews, 11,* CD010013.

Mayo Clinic Center for Social Media (2012). *Bringing the Social Media #Revolution to Healthcare.* Rochester, MN: Mayo Foundation for Medical Education & Research.

Merchant, R.M., Elmer, S., & Lurie, N. (2011). Integrating social media into emergency preparedness efforts. *New England Journal of Medicine, 365*(4), 289–291.

Moorhead, S.A., Hazlett, D.E., Harrison, L., Carroll, J.K., Irwin, A., & Hoving, C. (2013). A new dimension of health care: Systematic review of the uses, benefits and limitations of social media for health communication. *Journal of Medical Internet Research, 15*(4), e85.

Moreno, M.A., Goniu, N., Moreno, P.S., & Diekema, D. (2013). Ethics of social media research: Common concerns and practical considerations. *Cyberpsychology, Behavior and Social Networking, 16*(9), 708–13.

Muessig, K.E., Pike, E.C., Legrand, S., & Hightow-Weidman, L.B. (2013). Mobile phone applications for the care and prevention of HIV and other sexually transmitted diseases: A review. *Journal of Medical Internet Research, 15,* e1.

O'Connor, D. (2013). The apomediated world: Regulation research when social media has changed research. *Journal of Law Medicine and Ethics, 41*(2), 470–483.

Pal, B.R. (2014). Social media for diabetes health education – Inclusive or exclusive? *Current Diabetes Reviews, 10,* 284–290.

Ramo, D.E., & Prochaska, J. (2012). Broad reach and targeted recruitment using Facebook for an online survey of young adult substance use. *Journal of Medical Internet Research, 14,* e28.

Schuchman, M. (2014). The promise and pitfalls of global mHealth. *Canadian Medical Association Journal, 186*(15), 1134–1135.

Secretary's Advisory Committee on Human Research Protections (SACHRP) (2013). *Considerations and recommendations concerning internet research and human subjects research regulations, with revisions.* Retrieved from http://www.hhs.gov/ohrp/sachrp/commsec/attachmentbsecletter20.pdf

Stephens, S.W., Williams, C., Gray, R., Kerby, J.D., & Wang, H.E. (2013). Preliminary experience with social media for community consultation and public disclosure in exception from informed consent trials. *Circulation, 128*(3), 267–270.

Thomas, J.C., Sage, M., Dillenberg, J., & Guillory, V.J. (2002). A code of ethics for public health. *American Journal of Public Health, 92*(7), 1057–1059.

Thompson, B.M., & Brodsky, I. (2013). Should the FDA regulate mobile medical apps? *BMJ, 347,* f5211.

Thompson, L.A., Black, E., Duff, W.P., Paradise Black, N., Saliba, H., & Dawson, K. (2011). Protected health information on social networking sites: Ethical and legal considerations. *Journal of Medical Internet Research, 13,* e9.

Tweet, M.S., Gulati, R., Aase, L.A., & Hayes, S.N. (2011). Spontaneous coronary artery dissection: A disease-specific, social networking community-initiated study. *Mayo Clinic Proceedings, 86*(9), 845–850.

Vayena, E., Mastroianni, A., & Kahn, J. (2012). Ethical issues in health research with novel online sources. *American Journal of Public Health, 102*(12), 2225–2230.

Vayena, E., Mastroianni, A., & Kahn, J. (2013). Caught in the web: Informed consent for online health research. *Science Translational Medicine, 5*(173), 173fs6.

Vayena, E., & Tasioulas, J. (2013). Adapting standards: Ethical oversight of participant-led health research. *PLoS Medicine, 10*(3), e1001401.

Velasco, E., Agheneza, T., Denecke, K., Kirchner, G., & Eckmanns, T. (2014). Social media and internet-based data in global systems for public health surveillance: A systematic review. *Milbank Quarterly, 92,* 7–33.

Vital Wave Consulting. (2009). *mHealth for Development: The Opportunity of Mobile Technology for Healthcare in the Developing World.* Washington, D.C. and Newbury, UK: UN Foundation–Vodafone Foundation Partnership.

Wicks, P., Vaughan, T.E., Massagli, M.P., & Heywood, J. (2011). Accelerated clinical discovery using self-reported patient data collected online and a patient-matching algorithm. *Nature Biotechnology, 29,* 411–414.

World Bank. (2012). *Information and Communications for Development: Maximizing Mobile.* Washington DC: World Bank.

Weitzman, E.R., Adida, B., Kelemen, S., & Mandl, K.D. (2011). Sharing data for public health research by members of an international online diabetes social network. *PLoS One, 6*(4), e19256.

Zickuhr, K., & Smith, A. (2012). *Digital Differences. Pew Internet and American Life Project.* Washington, DC: Pew Charitable Trusts.

Online professionalism: A synthetic review

KATHERINE C. CHRETIEN & MATTHEW G. TUCK

VA Medical Center, Washington, DC and George Washington University School of Medicine and Health Sciences, Washington DC, USA

Abstract

The rise of social media has increased connectivity and blurred personal and professional boundaries, bringing new challenges for medical professionalism. Whether traditional professionalism principles apply to the online social media space remains unknown. The purpose of this synthetic literature review was to characterize the original peer-reviewed research studies published between 1 January 2000–1 November 2014 on online professionalism, to assess methodologies and approaches used, and to provide insights to guide future studies in this area. The investigators searched three databases and performed manual searches of bibliographies to identify the 32 studies included. Most studies originated in the USA. Cross-sectional surveys and analyses of publicly available online content were the most common methodologies employed. Studies covered the general areas of use and privacy, assessment of unprofessional online behaviours, consensus-gathering of what constitutes unprofessional or inappropriate online behaviours, and education and policies. Studies were of variable quality; only around half of survey studies had response rates of 50% or greater. Medical trainees were the most common population studied. Future directions for research include public perspectives of online professionalism, impact on patient trust, and how to use social media productively as medical professionals.

Introduction

Over the last decade, the world has witnessed exponential growth of social media. In 2004 the social networking site Facebook was started at Harvard College. The site, as of 2014, boasted over 1 billion users worldwide (Facebook, 2014). Other social media platforms are also rising, albeit at different rates, while others have fallen; yet the overall trend of greater adoption and connectivity stands (Lunden, 2013).

This increased connectivity and blurring of personal and professional boundaries on social media has introduced new challenges for medical professionalism. Social media has allowed the public greater access to potentially intimate details of their healthcare providers' lives. Physicians' characters have been judged by their online actions, and momentary slips in judgement have had lasting consequences (Greysen et al., 2010).

While many definitions for medical professionalism exist, most include commitments to professional competence, integrity, patient confidentiality, patient welfare and social justice; upholding these commitments is considered the basis for public trust (ABIM Foundation et al., 2002). Recent attempts have been made to apply these traditional principles to the online setting through the issuance of national guidelines and policies for physicians' social media use (Farnan et al., 2013; Shore et al., 2011). The intersection between medical professionalism and social media has been termed online professionalism, also called e-professionalism or digital professionalism (Cain & Romanelli, 2009; Ellaway & Tworek, 2011; Greysen et al., 2010). Whether traditional professionalism principles apply to the online social media space remains unknown – a space where there may be disinhibiting anonymity, indistinct personal and professional boundaries, potential for rapid dissemination and amplification of content, and an ever-present and sometimes unclear audience.

Prior reviews have focused on the use of social media in medical education (Cheston et al., 2013) and qualitative textual analysis of social media's professionalism challenges and opportunities (Gholami-Kordkheili et al., 2013). The purpose of this synthetic literature review is to explore the field of online professionalism by characterizing the original peer-reviewed research studies published to date, to assess methodologies and approaches used, and to provide insights to guide future studies in this area.

Methods

Our focus was on peer-reviewed original research studies that addressed online professionalism of medical students, residents, or physicians. We searched

PubMed, CINAHL and Google Scholar for publications in English since 1 January 2000 to 1 November 2014 using the terms 'professionalism AND (social media OR Internet)' in any field, yielding 941 titles. Two investigators independently performed the searches and subsequent title and abstract review to identify candidate publications for full-text review. We also performed a manual search of bibliographies of included papers. We excluded commentaries, reviews, evaluation of educational curricula to teach online professionalism, and studies exclusively involving other health professionals. One study was excluded because it was too closely related to another included study to contribute additional insights. The two independent lists of studies to include were compared and discrepancies were resolved through discussion.

Once the included list of papers was finalized, one investigator (K.C.) abstracted the date of publication, the date the study was performed, methodology, target population, country of origin, key measures, limitations, ethical statement, and miscellaneous notes. The second investigator (M.T.) reviewed and confirmed the data abstraction. Based on review and inductive coding of key measures, four main themes of study emerged.

Results

We included 32 studies in the review (Table 1). The earliest publication year was 2008, with two studies published. Only one study was published in 2009. Following this year, there was sustained level of activity in this area: six in 2010, five in 2011, seven in 2012, six in 2013, five in 2014. Note, 2014 does not include studies published in the final 2 months. Most studies were based in the USA (25, 78%). Other study sites were based in the UK (2, 6%), Canada (2, 6%), Brazil (1, 3%), France (1, 3%), and New Zealand (1, 3%). Two of the US studies involved analysis of social media content or profiles from multiple countries (Chretien et al., 2011a; Lagu et al., 2008).

Most commonly used methodologies were cross-sectional surveys (19, 59%) and analysis of publicly available Internet content such as Facebook profiles, Twitter streams, or blogs (11; 34%). Other methods used included focus groups, mixed-methods involving individual interviews followed by survey, and one experimental study. Of note, of the many survey studies, only about half had response rates of 50% or greater, and three survey studies either did not explicitly report a response rate or stated they could not calculate one (Jain et al., 2014; Osman et al., 2012; Rocha & de Castro, 2014). For the 11 studies that analysed publicly available Internet content, four (36%) did not mention any methods to increase study

rigour of data extraction and analysis expected of content analyses such as having multiple reviewers or extractors and achieving acceptable inter-rater reliability (Landman et al., 2010; Langenfeld et al., 2014; MacDonald et al., 2010; Thompson et al., 2008).

Study populations often involved medical trainees, with 25 (78%) involving medical students and/or resident physicians and fellows. Twelve studies (38%) included medical educators or medical school administrators. Other studies involved practising physicians (6; 19%), laypersons (2; 6%), or medical school websites (1, 3%).

Most studies included (31; 97%) had clear ethical statements within the paper either stating ethical board approval, exemption, or determination that ethical approval was not necessary. Of the 11 studies that performed analysis on publicly available data on the Internet, including individual Facebook profiles, six (55%) were found to meet criteria for institutional review board exemption, three (27%) were approved, and one did not have an ethical statement published. In addition, one study's authors noted in their methods that they did not seek ethical approval due to the public nature of the data, however pursued retroactive ethical approval as a result of editorial suggestion (MacDonald et al., 2010).

In terms of themes covered in the studies, there were several major areas that the studies addressed: use and privacy, assessment of unprofessional behaviour, consensus gathering, and education and policies.

Use and privacy

Studies that asked medical trainees, medical educators and practising physicians about their own social networking use found highest use among trainees, with medical student use being highest in general (Black et al., 2010; Garner & O Sullivan, 2010; Ginory et al., 2012; Moubarak et al., 2011; Thompson et al., 2008; White et al., 2013). Lower rates of use were seen in medical education faculty staff (Barker et al., 2012; Chretien et al., 2011b; Jain et al., 2014; Kesselheim et al., 2014; Kind et al., 2012; Patel et al., 2012). Practising physicians were closer in usage to medical education faculty staff (Bosslet et al., 2011).

Thompson et al. (2008) were the first to report the use of privacy settings on Facebook accounts of medical trainees. In their study, only a minority (38%) enabled privacy settings. Subsequent studies showed higher rates of privacy setting deployment from 50–93% among residency applicants, residents, and physicians (Garner & O'Sullivan, 2010; Ginory et al., 2012; Koh et al., 2013; Landman et al., 2010; MacDonald et al., 2010; Moubarak et al., 2011; Osman et al., 2012), including a later cohort of medical

Table 1. Studies of online professionalism included in literature review.

Study	Methodology	Date study performed	Target population	Country of origin	Key measures	Ethics statement
Thompson et al., 2008	Analysis of Facebook profiles; in-depth analysis of 10 randomly selected profiles	2007	501 medical students, 312 residents at a single institution	USA	Presence of profile, privacy settings, personal information, groups, photo content	Yes; Exempt
Lagu et al., 2008	Content analysis of blogs	2006	271 medical blogs written by doctors or nurses	USA*	Blog content, characteristics, patient portrayals, patient privacy violations, unprofessional content	Not found
Chretien et al., 2009	Survey, RR 60%	2009	78 deans of student affairs or their proxies at US medical schools	USA	Percentage of schools reporting incidents of students posting unprofessional content online, type of professionalism infraction, disciplinary actions taken, existence of institution policies, and plans for policy development	Yes; Approved
Kind et al., 2010	Analysis of medical school websites	2010	132 LCME accredited US medical schools	USA	Medical school presence on social media sites, publicly available policies on online social networking	Yes; Exempt
Black et al., 2010	Analysis of Facebook profiles	2007, 2009	528 medical students, 712 residents at a single institution	USA	Presence of profile, privacy settings, personally identifiable information, photo content, group membership, information not usually disclosed in a doctor–patient encounter	Yes; Exempt
Garner & O'Sullivan, 2010	Survey, RR 31%	2009	56 medical students	UK	Facebook usage, privacy settings, groups membership related to course, professional behaviours	Yes; Approved
MacDonald et al., 2010	Analysis of Facebook profiles	2008	338 doctors graduated in 2006 and 2007 from a single institution	New Zealand	Facebook membership, privacy settings utilization, content revealed	Yes; Retroactively approved
Chretien et al., 2010	Focus groups	2009	64 medical students at a single institution	US	Online habits, nature of students' postings, what would constitute inappropriate posted material, perspectives on institutional guidelines	Yes; Approved
Landman et al., 2010	Analysis of Facebook profiles	2009	127 general surgery faculty staff and 88 residents at a single institution	USA	Presence of profile, privacy settings, work-related postings, unprofessional content	Yes; Exempt
Thompson et al., 2011	Analysis of Facebook profiles	2007, 2009	1023 medical students and residents with Facebook profiles at a single institution	USA	Protected health information in text or photos within Facebook profiles	Yes; Exempt

(Continued)

Table 1. (*Continued*)

Study	Methodology	Date study performed	Target population	Country of origin	Key measures	Ethics statement
Moubarak et al., 2011	Survey, RR 50%	2009	202 residents and fellows at a single institution	France	SNS use, privacy settings, opinions on the effect of SNS use and the doctor–patient relationship	Yes; Approved
Chretien et al., 2011a	Content analysis of tweets and Twitter profiles	2010	260 physicians on Twitter, 5156 tweets	USA[a]	Descriptive elements of profiles including identifiability, speciality, geographic location, content of tweets, unprofessional tweets	Yes; Approved
Bosslet et al., 2011	Survey, RR 16%	2010	335 medical students, residents, practising physicians national sample)	USA	Social networking site use, percentage receiving friend requests, acceptance of friend requests, attitudes towards use and patient interactions	Yes; Approved
Chretien et al., 2011b	Survey, RR 75%	2010	82 internal medicine clerkship directors (national sample)	USA	Social networking site use, professional boundaries and friending, appropriateness of hypothetical student-posted content	Yes; Ethical approval not required
Ginory et al., 2012	Survey, RR 29%	2011	182 psychiatry residents (national sample)	USA	Facebook use, privacy settings, information disclosed on profiles, friend requests, searching for patients on Facebook, and concerns of use, and knowledge of any incidents	Yes; Exempt
Osman et al., 2012	Survey, no RR available	Not stated	42 students, 20 first year doctors, 20 senior doctors at a single institution	UK	Facebook use, publicly accessible material, awareness of privacy guidelines and online professionalism	Yes; Ethical approval determined not required
Patel et al., 2012	Survey, RR 96% for residents 81% for students, 80% for faculty members	Not stated	16 medical education faculty, 120 first-year residents, 130 third-year medical students at a single institution	USA	Usage, attitudes, instructional preferences	Yes; Approved
Greysen et al., 2012	Survey, RR 71%	2011	68 executive directors of state medical boards (national sample)	USA	Incidence of online professionalism violations and type, how reported, any disciplinary actions taken	Yes; Approved
Kind et al., 2012	Survey, RR 65%	2010	94 paediatric clerkship directors (national sample)	USA	Social networking site use, friend requests, ratings of hypothetical online content by students	Yes; Approved
Golden et al., 2012	Analysis of Facebook profiles	2011	234 applicants to ENT residency programme at a single institution	USA	Presence of profile, publicly accessible information, professionalism score	Yes; Approved

(*Continued*)

Table 1. (*Continued*)

Study	Methodology	Date study performed	Target population	Country of origin	Key measures	Ethics statement
Barker et al., 2012	Survey, RR 50%	2010	132 anaesthesiology programme directors (national sample)	USA	Presence of social networking policies and educational programmes, incidents of reprimand due to inappropriate social networking use, utilization of social networking by programme directors both personally and for resident background searches	Yes; Exempt
White et al., 2013	Mixed methods: interviews followed by survey RR 17%	2011	14 health professional students (6 medical students) for individual interviews; 682 health professional students (232 medical students) at a single institution	Canada	Facebook use, what constitutes unprofessional posted content	Yes; Approved
Greysen et al., 2013	Survey, RR 71%	2011	68 executive directors of state medical boards (national sample)	USA	Likelihood of investigating 10 hypothetical vignettes involving physicians' posted content	Yes; Approved
Koh et al., 2013	Survey, RR 84%	2010	178 members of the Group on Advancement of Psychiatry, from trainees to retired (national sample)	USA	Use of social media and e-mail, posting online information, restricting information, searching patient information online	Yes; Exempt
Ponce et al., 2013	Analysis of Facebook profiles	2010	431 medical student applicants to 2010 orthopaedic residency match at a single institution	USA	Unprofessional content, privacy settings, USMLE Step 1 score, age, residency applicant composite score	Yes; Approved
Ross et al., 2013	Survey, RR 34%	Not stated	236 medical students at single institution	Canada	Understanding of professionalism and perceptions of professionalism in online environments	Yes; Approved
Cook et al., 2013	Survey, RR 61%	2012	122 categorical paediatric residency programme directors (national sample)	USA	Structure of ethics and professionalism curricula, methods of assessment, use of resources and social media policies	Yes; Approved
Clyde et al., 2014	Experimental	Not stated	250 'public' participants, mostly college students at a single institution	USA	First Impressions of Medical Professionalism scale developed for the study, used with experimental Facebook profiles (strictly professional, personal/healthy; personal unhealthy)	Yes; Approved

(*Continued*)

Table 1. (*Continued*)

Study	Methodology	Date study performed	Target population	Country of origin	Key measures	Ethics statement
Jain et al., 2014	Survey, no RR available	2009	1421 medical students, faculty staff and the public (non-health professional staff) at a single institution	USA	Appropriateness ratings on staged screenshots of medical students, comfort on having student as their future doctor	Yes; Exempt
Kesselheim et al., 2014)	Survey, RR 33%	2011	162 paediatric programme directors and associate programme directors (national sample)	USA	Social networking site use, appropriateness ratings of resident social networking use (friending, accessing during work), experience with inappropriate resident behaviour, policy, and education	Yes; Approved
Rocha & de Castro, 2014	Survey, RR not explicitly stated	Not stated	350 medical students at a single institution	Brazil	Opinions on potential repercussion of posts by medical students and doctors, how often students came across 10 examples of unprofessional behaviour, rate appropriateness of examples	Yes; Approved
Langenfeld et al., 2014	Analysis of Facebook profiles	Not stated	319 accessible Facebook profiles of surgical residents (regional sample)	USA	Incidence of professional, potentially unprofessional, and clearly unprofessional content	Yes; Exempt

RR, Response rate; SNS, social networking site; USMLE, United States Medical Licensing Examination.
[a]Study included data from international sources.

trainees at the same institution of the initial Thompson study (Black et al., 2010).

Assessment of unprofessional behaviour

Many studies have tried to assess to what degree medical professionals are posting unprofessional content online. These used either survey or content analysis methodologies. Surveys captured medical students' self-report and medical educators' or administrators' experiences encountering unprofessional incidents by those under their supervision. When medical students were surveyed in the UK and Canada they reported seeing unprofessional behaviour by their colleagues on sites such as Facebook (44–88%) to a higher degree than how they self-reported their own behaviour (Garner & O'Sullivan, 2010; Osman et al., 2012; White et al., 2013). Brazilian medical students reported witnessing all examples of unprofessional online behaviour by other medical students or physicians presented to them, from patient privacy violations (14%), to sexual or sexually

suggestive content (42%), to photos suggesting alcohol intoxication (74%), to pictures in a bathing suit (83%) (Rocha & de Castro, 2014). While the authors deemed pictures in a bathing suit to be unprofessional, students rated them neutral in appropriateness (Rocha & de Castro, 2014).

Surveys of medical educators and administrators confirmed that incidents involving unprofessional content online by medical professionals have reached the attention of medical leadership and have at times resulted in serious consequences (Barker et al., 2012; Chretien et al., 2009; Greysen et al., 2012; Kesselheim et al., 2014). In a national sample of deans of students affairs of US medical schools, 60% reported ever having incidents of unprofessional content posted by students at their institutions (Chretien et al., 2009). Three incidents had resulted in dismissal from medical school (Chretien et al., 2009). Paediatric residency programme directors and associate programme directors encountered residents posting inappropriate comments about hospital staff most frequently, followed by inappropriate comments about patients, self, and workplace (Kesselheim et al., 2014). About a third (34%) had counselled one to three residents in social networking site (SNS)-related lapses in professionalism in the past year (Kesselheim et al., 2014). Approximately 18% of anaesthesiology programme directors have had to reprimand a resident or fellow for online professionalism issues (Barker et al., 2012). Greysen and colleagues surveyed executive directors of US state medical boards responsible for the licensing of practising physicians and found that 92% had ever had at least one of several online professionalism violations reported to their boards (Greysen et al., 2012). The most common reported violations were inappropriate patient communication online, use of the Internet for inappropriate practice, and online misrepresentation of credentials (Greysen et al., 2012). The majority of boards held formal disciplinary proceedings in response to violations, with some outcomes including license suspension, restriction or revocation (Greysen et al., 2012).

Other studies approached assessment of unprofessional online behaviour through direct evaluation of posted online content. Review of Facebook profiles was a common approach taken (Black et al., 2010; Golden et al., 2012; Landman et al., 2010; Langenfeld et al., 2014; MacDonald et al., 2010; Ponce et al., 2013; Thompson et al., 2008, 2011).

Evaluation of Twitter feeds (Chretien et al., 2011a) and blogs (Lagu et al., 2008) was also performed. In all of these studies, the processes used to determine what constituted unprofessional content varied. Some relied on consensus of two or more reviewers (Chretien et al., 2011a); some created novel scoring or categorization systems but were still largely subjective (Golden et al., 2012; Langenfeld et al., 2014; Ponce et al., 2013). Others reported frequencies of encountering specific examples of content such as depicted intoxication, profanity, or patient descriptions (Lagu et al., 2008; Landman et al., 2010; MacDonald et al., 2010; Thompson et al., 2008). One study reported that all (12) patient privacy violations found within trainees' public Facebook profiles involved photos from medical mission trips (Thompson et al., 2011).

Consensus gathering

What is unprofessional online behaviour? Studies have examined the perceptions of stakeholders in order to help determine consensus around what constitutes unprofessional online behaviour. Stakeholders have included health profession students, medical educators, and laypersons.

Aside from patient privacy violations and illegal activity, studies involving medical students often failed to establish agreed definitions of unprofessional or inappropriate online behaviour (Chretien et al., 2010; Ross et al., 2013; White et al., 2013). Some students felt that nothing was 'inappropriate', and what they chose to post on their personal time was distinct and divorced from their 8:00 a.m. to 5:00 p.m. professional selves (Chretien et al., 2010; Ross et al., 2013). Medical students did not always believe that they are held to a higher standard (Chretien et al., 2010; Ross et al., 2013).

A number of surveys asked respondents to rate hypothetical online postings on the appropriateness of the behaviours in order to find consensus. Table 2 shows key findings of six of these studies, with the specific behaviours studied listed from most inappropriate to least inappropriate as rated by survey respondents, placed in rank order for each study based on reported data (Chretien et al., 2011b; Greysen et al., 2013; Jain et al., 2014; Kesselheim et al., 2014; Kind et al., 2012; Rocha & de Castro, 2014). Of these studies, one found that younger medical educator respondents were less likely to deem the behaviours inappropriate across all cases, although this did not reach statistical significance (Chretien et al., 2011b). Most hypothetical postings were drawn from prior studies identifying potential unprofessional content within medical professionals' social media pages (Lagu et al., 2008; Thompson et al., 2008) as well as the authors' own experiences. Note that the Greysen et al. (2013) study involved surveying the executive directors of US state medical boards who are responsible for the licensing of all US physicians. The hypothetical vignettes were chosen after consultation with key informants in order to identify the online physician behaviours most concerning to boards in terms of protecting the public. Across the studies, multiple stakeholder groups found patient privacy violations, patient content in general, sexually suggestive or explicit material and negative comments about faculty staff, colleagues, and institution to be the most unprofessional (Table 2).

Only two studies to date have attempted to gather perspectives of the public, or at least a defined subset of the public. One study surveyed laypersons (non-doctor, non-student employees of a university), medical students, and faculty members at one institution (Jain et al., 2014). In response to screenshots of Facebook profiles of medical students that were created for the study, respondents rated each screenshot for appropriateness and comfort level of having the student as their future doctor. Faculty members and the non-health professional employees were more conservative than students on the appropriateness of the content, and faculty members had even higher expectations for students than laypersons. Of note, the sample of non-health professional employees was fairly

Table 2. The most inappropriate to least inappropriate online behaviours in six studies of online professionalism.

Study	Rocha & de Castro, 2014	Chretien et al., 2011b	Kind et al., 2012	Greysen et al., 2013	Kesselheim et al., 2014	Jain et al., 2014
Population	Medical students in Brazil at one institution	National sample of internal medicine clerkship directors in the USA	National sample of paediatric clerkship directors in the USA	Executive directors of US state medical boards	National sample of paediatric programme directors and associate programme directors in the USA	Faculty members, medical students, and non-health professional university employees at one institution in the USA
Hypothetical cases posted by	Medical students	Medical students	Medical students	Physicians	Residents	Medical students
Most inappropriate[a]	Patient privacy violation; Negative comments about patients; Negative comments about medical school, colleagues or doctors; Sexual or sexually suggestive content	Sexually explicit material; Discriminatory language; Profanity; Depicted intoxication; Negative comments about faculty; Negative comments about institution; Description of de-identified patient encounter using negative tone; Negative comments about medical profession; Photo of student with alcohol	Discriminatory language; Sexually explicit material; Negative comments about faculty; Profanity; Description of de-identified patient encounter using negative tone; Depicted intoxication; Negative comments about institution; Negative comments about profession	Misleading information about clinical outcomes; Posting patient images without consent; Mis-representation of credentials; Inappropriate patient contact	Posting content about patients; Friending patients; Negative comments about the workplace	Negative comments about patients; Image with marijuana
Moderately inappropriate[b]	Negative comments about profession; Depicted intoxication; Photos depicting alcohol consumption	Description of de-identified patient encounter using respectful tone	Photo of student with alcohol; Description of de-identified patient encounter using respectful tone	Depicted intoxication; Breach of patient confidentiality; Discriminatory speech about patients	Access SNS profiles of residency applicants	Partial nudity; Description or depiction of clinical scenario in US; Same-sex pairs posting together or kissing; Depiction of clinical scenario in international setting; Image with alcohol; Image with cigarettes
Least inappropriate[c]	Pictures in bathing suit			Derogatory speech about patients; Photos of alcohol use without intoxication; Patient narratives without privacy violations		Images of parties and dancing; Comments on medical school; Opposite-sex pairs posing together or kissing

[a]Items with >75% agreement or study equivalent.
[b]Items with 50–75% agreement or study equivalent.
[c]Items with <50% agreement or study equivalent.

homogeneous, being predominantly white, female with a mean age of 40.8 years (Jain et al., 2014).

The other study that targeted public perspectives on online professionalism was an experimental study that randomly assigned 'potential patients' (mainly college students) to view staged physician Facebook profiles that contained either strictly professional content, personal content that was healthy (e.g. hiking, reading), or personal material that was unhealthy (e.g. over-eating, sleeping in) (Clyde et al. , 2014). Participants then rated each physician on a professionalism scale developed for the study. Clyde et al. found that profiles with healthy personal content were rated as the most professional, even more so than profiles with strictly professional content (Clyde et al., 2014).

What are appropriate professional boundaries on social networking sites?

Survey studies of medical educators have investigated appropriate boundaries between faculty, trainees, and colleagues terms of 'friending,' or connecting, on SNS (Chretien et al., 2011b; Kesselheim et al., 2014; Kind et al., 2012). In general, educators felt it was inappropriate to become SNS friends with current supervisees or learners, but more acceptable with former supervisees or learners. A group of health professional students, including medical students, reported low rates of being connected to current instructors (5%) but higher rates with former instructors (21%) (White et al., 2013). In addition, there was consensus that friending colleagues on SNS was appropriate online behaviour (Chretien et al., 2011b; Kesselheim et al., 2014; Kind et al., 2012).

In terms of connecting with patients on SNS, there is high consensus among medical educators that it is inappropriate to become SNS friends with current patients (Chretien et al., 2011b; Kesselheim et al., 2014; Kind et al., 2012). A 2010 random, stratified mail survey of US medical students, resident physicians and practising physicians also looked at friend requests by patients or patients' family members and found that practising physicians were more likely to receive requests (35%) than residents (8%) or students (1%) (Bosslet et al., 2011). Respondents very rarely requested to be a SNS friend with a patient or a patient's family member (1%). Overall, respondents did not think it was ethical to interact with patients within social networking sites whether for social or patient-care reasons, and were concerned about the ability to maintain patient confidentiality on social media platforms (Bosslet et al., 2011).

Studies have also investigated whether psychiatrists and psychiatry residents look up their patients online for collateral information for their care or otherwise (Ginory et al., 2012; Koh et al., 2013).

A survey of psychiatric residents found that 19% had looked up patient information online (Ginory et al., 2012), and in a mixed sample of academic psychiatrists, 35% reported doing so (Koh et al., 2013). In addition, one study asked anaesthesia residency programme directors whether they searched for applicant or resident information online, and 42% reported such use at least a few times (Barker et al., 2012).

Education and policies

Educational efforts and institutional policies have been another focus for studies of online professionalism. Existence and/or knowledge of social media professionalism policies or educational curricula designed to address online professionalism have been queried alongside assessment of incidents (Barker et al., 2012; Chretien et al., 2009; Kesselheim et al., 2014; Osman et al., 2012; Rocha & de Castro, 2014). Cook et al. (2013) surveyed categorical paediatric programme directors on instruction provided to trainees about professional behaviour on social media as well as their social media policies. Another study analysed medical school websites to find publicly accessible social media policies and main themes therein (Kind et al., 2010).

Patel and colleagues (2012) surveyed medical students, residents and faculty staff on their social media use, attitudes and instructional preferences in order to identify who best should mentor students in professional social media use. While residents were more similar to students in usage patterns and preference for mentoring techniques, residents did not feel as prepared to mentor students without additional guidance as compared with faculty members (Patel et al., 2012).

Discussion

Since the initial studies in 2008, there has been sustained research activity in the area of online professionalism. In general, surveys and analysis of publicly available online content have been the preferred methodologies. Major areas of focus have included use and privacy, assessment of unprofessional behaviour, consensus gathering on what constitutes unprofessional behaviour and appropriate professional boundaries, and education and policy.

Compared to other literature reviews published on related topics, this review is the first to synthesize original research in online professionalism in terms of methods, subjects, and themes. Gholami-Kordkheili and colleagues (2013) performed a qualitative systematic review on the challenges and opportunities social media created for medical professionalism. They included original research, commentaries and editorials published between 2002–2011 and performed qualitative text analysis to result in 10 social media-related opportunities and 13 social media challenges (Gholami-Kordkheili et al., 2013). Another systematic review addressed social media use in medical education, with the 14 studies included involving social media as educational interventions (Cheston et al., 2013). One challenge cited in using social media as an education tool was concern about privacy and security, although the possibility for promotion of professional development was seen as an opportunity (Cheston et al., 2013).

While the published body of literature has grown quickly over the last 6 years, the quality of studies is variable. Many of the survey studies had low or unclear response rates. Also, while some authors applied rigorous analysis techniques to the examination of online content, including multiple independent reviewers and formal calculation of inter-rater reliability, there were also many studies in which the methods were vague, unclear and lacking rigour. Six (19%) publications did not disclose which time frame the studies were conducted in. As studies could ask for time-sensitive conditions such as social media use and existence of policy, lack of time frame is especially problematic. It is unclear whether the low quality of some published studies is a factor of editorial interest in this emerging topic, or simply a general comment on educational research publication. In the systematic review on social media in medical education, the Medical Education Research Study Quality Instrument scores calculated reflected the low to moderate quality of studies included (Cheston et al., 2013).

Ethical questions arose among the subset of studies included that assessed publicly available online content, such as Facebook profiles. Notably, in one study that examined Facebook profiles of new physicians, the authors specifically mentioned that they did not feel any ethical approval was necessary due to the public nature of the data and did not pursue ethical body approval prior to submitting the study for publication (MacDonald et al., 2010). Upon editorial suggestion after submission, they sought and were granted retroactive ethical approval, and discussed their considerations within the paper. We could not locate the ethical approval of another study that analysed blog content (Lagu et al., 2008). Another study that employed survey methods to assess Facebook use, publicly accessible material and awareness of privacy guidelines in students and doctors, noted in their abstract, 'It was an ethical risk to access publicly available information online as many users do not appreciate the lack of privacy involved, therefore a cross-sectional survey was undertaken' page e549 (Osman et al., 2012). The ethical issues involved in performing Internet-based research are

many and have been written about by others (Eysenbach & Till, 2001). Public versus private spaces, informed consent, and potential for harm need consideration(Eysenbach & Till, 2001).

In general, the studies included in this review focus on unprofessional behaviour, whether in its assessment, interpretation, education, or boundary lines. This reflects how the field of 'online professionalism' has evolved. A broader definition of professionalism includes positive behaviours and thus 'online professionalism' could also include studies of how medical professionals and trainees use social media in professionally rewarding ways, capitalizing on the opportunities afforded by social media such as providing expert advice on health matters to society (ABIM Foundation et al., 2002; Greysen et al., 2010). Future reviews might focus on these studies that might not be categorized under 'professionalism' but might be found through different search terms such as 'meaningful use'.

When assessing whether content was unprofessional, studies differed in terms of standards and processes used. This reflects a key challenge with future research in this area as studies often rely upon subjective assessments, either on the part of the researchers or of the study subjects. Indeed, age appears to influence perceptions of behaviour, let alone other individual background or cultural influences. Standards for online professionalism may be evolving. The work in consensus gathering has helped contribute to our understanding of how various groups view online professionalism. The similarities and differences identified therein can inform our approaches to teaching, assessment, and policy-making.

In this vein, other opportunities for future study include additional public perspectives of online professionalism beyond the small defined populations studied to date – particularly minorities, those of lower social economic status, and those with lower technology use. How is patient trust impacted by displays of physician-posted content? In addition, studies that elucidate how social media can be used productively as medical professionals (for career advancement, to help patients individually or collectively) are greatly needed.

This review has limitations. The search study employed was limited did not include terms such as 'social networking' and 'ethics'. As above, it may not have captured studies of positive social media use. However, we included a manual search of bibliographies of included papers and also searched three separate databases that yielded a robust number of studies.

In conclusion, the body of literature representing online professionalism continues to grow. Care must be taken to produce high quality studies that carefully consider ethical issues related to

Internet-based research, that factor in the subjective influences within the field, and add to our existing knowledge. These studies can help guide our navigation of digital space as we only grow further connected with time.

Declaration of interest: The authors report no conflicts of interest. The authors alone are responsible for the content and writing of the paper.

References

ABIM Foundation (American Board of Internal Medicine, ACP-ASIM Foundation. American College of Physicians, American Society of Internal Medicine, & European Federation of Internal Medicine). (2002). Medical professionalism in the new millennium: A physician charter. *Annals of Internal Medicine*, *136*(3), 243–246.

Barker, A.L., Wehbe-Janek, H., Bhandari, N.S., Bittenbinder, T.M., Jo, C., & McAllister, R.K. (2012). A national cross-sectional survey of social networking practices of U.S. anesthesiology residency program directors. *Journal of Clinical Anesthesia*, *24*(8), 618–624. doi:10.1016/j.jclinane.2012.06.002

Black, E.W., Thompson, L.A., Duff, W.P., Dawson, K., Saliba, H., & Black, N.M.P. (2010). Revisiting social network utilization by physicians-in-training. *Journal of Graduate Medical Education*, *2*(2), 289–293. doi:10.4300/JGME-D-10-00011.1

Bosslet, G.T., Torke, A.M., Hickman, S.E., Terry, C.L., & Helft, P.R. (2011). The patient–doctor relationship and online social networks: Results of a national survey. *Journal of General Internal Medicine*, *26*(10), 1168–1174. doi:10.1007/s11606-011-1761-2

Cain, J., & Romanelli, F. (2009). E-professionalism: A new paradigm for a digital age. *Currents in Pharmacy Teaching and Learning*, *1*(2), 66–70. doi:10.1016/j.cptl.2009.10.001

Cheston, C.C., Flickinger, T.E., & Chisolm, M.S. (2013). Social media use in medical education: A systematic review. *Academic Medicine*, *88*(6), 893–901. doi:10.1097/ACM.0b013e31828ffc23

Chretien, K.C., Azar, J., & Kind, T. (2011a). Physicians on Twitter. *Journal of the American Medical Association*, *305*(6), 566–568. doi:10.1001/jama.2011.68

Chretien, K.C., Farnan, J.M., Greysen, S.R., & Kind, T. (2011b). To friend or not to friend? Social networking and faculty perceptions of online professionalism. *Academic Medicine*, *86*(12), 1545–1550. doi:10.1097/ACM.0b013e3182356128

Chretien, K.C., Goldman, E.F., Beckman, L., & Kind, T. (2010). It's your own risk: medical students' perspectives on online professionalism. *Academic Medicine*, *85*(Suppl.10), S68–71. doi:10.1097/ACM.0b013e3181ed4778

Chretien, K.C., Greysen, S.R., Chretien, J.-P., & Kind, T. (2009). Online posting of unprofessional content by medical students. *Journal of the American Medical Association*, *302*(12), 1309–1315. doi:10.1001/jama.2009.1387

Clyde, J.W., Domenech Rodríguez, M.M., & Geiser, C. (2014). Medical professionalism: An experimental look at physicians' Facebook profiles. *Medical Education Online*, *19*, 23149.

Cook, A.F., Sobotka, S.A., & Ross, L.F. (2013). Teaching and assessment of ethics and professionalism: A survey of pediatric program directors. *Academic Pediatrics*, *13*(6), 570–576. doi:10.1016/j.acap.2013.07.009

Ellaway, R., & Tworek, J. (2011). Digital professionalism. Retrieved from https://www.aamc.org/members/gir/253674/viewpoint_july_11.html

Eysenbach, G., & Till, J.E. (2001). Ethical issues in qualitative research on Internet communities. *British Medical Journal*, *323*(7321), 1103–1105.

Facebook. (2014). Company Information. Retrieved from http://newsroom.fb.com/company-info/

Farnan, J.M., Snyder Sulmasy, L., Worster, B.K., Chaudhry, H.J., Rhyne, J.A., Arora, V.M., ... Federation of State Medical Boards Special Committee on Ethics and Professionalism. (2013). Online medical professionalism: Patient and public relationships: Policy statement from the American College of Physicians and the Federation of State Medical Boards. *Annals of Internal Medicine*, *158*(8), 620–627. doi:10.7326/0003-4819-158-8-201304160-00100

Garner, J., & O'Sullivan, H. (2010). Facebook and the professional behaviours of undergraduate medical students. *Clinical Teacher*, *7*(2), 112–115. doi:10.1111/j.1743-498X.2010.00356.x

Gholami-Kordkheili, F., Wild, V., & Strech, D. (2013). The impact of social media on medical professionalism: A systematic qualitative review of challenges and opportunities. *Journal of Medical Internet Research*, *15*(8), e184. doi:10.2196/jmir.2708

Ginory, A., Sabatier, L.M., & Eth, S. (2012). Addressing therapeutic boundaries in social networking. *Psychiatry*, *75*, 40–48. doi:10.1521/psyc.2012.75.1.40

Golden, J.B., Sweeny, L., Bush, B., & Carroll, W.R. (2012). Social networking and professionalism in otolaryngology residency applicants. *Laryngoscope*, *122*(7), 1493–1496. doi:10.1002/lary.23388

Greysen, S.R., Chretien, K.C., Kind, T., Young, A., & Gross, C.P. (2012). Physician violations of online professionalism and disciplinary actions: A national survey of state medical boards. *Journal of the American Medical Association*, *307*(11), 1141–1142. doi:10.1001/jama.2012.330

Greysen, S.R., Johnson, D., Kind, T., Chretien, K.C., Gross, C.P., Young, A., & Chaudhry, H.J. (2013). Online professionalism investigations by state medical boards: First, do no harm. *Annals of Internal Medicine*, *158*(2), 124–130. doi:10.7326/0003-4819-158-2-201301150-00008

Greysen, S.R., Kind, T., & Chretien, K.C. (2010). Online professionalism and the mirror of social media. *Journal of General Internal Medicine*, *25*(11), 1227–1229. doi:10.1007/s11606-010-1447-1

Jain, A., Petty, E.M., Jaber, R.M., Tackett, S., Purkiss, J., Fitzgerald, J., & White, C. (2014). What is appropriate to post on social media? Ratings from students, faculty members and the public. *Medical Education*, *48*(2), 157–169. doi:10.1111/medu.12282

Kesselheim, J.C., Batra, M., Belmonte, F., Boland, K.A., & McGregor, R.S. (2014). New professionalism challenges in medical training: An exploration of social networking. *Journal of Graduate Medical Education*, *6*, 100–105. doi:10.4300/JGME-D-13-00132.1

Kind, T., Genrich, G., Sodhi, A., & Chretien, K.C. (2010). Social media policies at US medical schools. *Medical Education Online*, *15*. doi:10.3402/meo.v15i0.5324

Kind, T., Greysen, S.R., & Chretien, K.C. (2012). Pediatric clerkship directors' social networking use and perceptions of online professionalism. *Academic Pediatrics*, *12*(2), 142–148. doi:10.1016/j.acap.2011.12.003

Koh, S., Cattell, G.M., Cochran, D.M., Krasner, A., Langheim, F.J.P., & Sasso, D.A. (2013). Psychiatrists' use of electronic communication and social media and a proposed framework for future guidelines. *Journal of Psychiatric Practice*, *19*(3), 254–263. doi:10.1097/01.pra.0000430511.90509.e2

Lagu, T., Kaufman, E.J., Asch, D.A., & Armstrong, K. (2008). Content of weblogs written by health professionals. *Journal of General Internal Medicine*, *23*(10), 1642–1646. doi:10.1007/s11606-008-0726-6

Landman, M.P., Shelton, J., Kauffmann, R.M., & Dattilo, J.B. (2010). Guidelines for maintaining a professional compass in the era of social networking. *Journal of Surgical Education*, *67*(6), 381–386. doi:10.1016/j.jsurg.2010.07.006

Langenfeld, S.J., Cook, G., Sudbeck, C., Luers, T., & Schenarts, P.J. (2014). An assessment of unprofessional behavior among surgical residents on Facebook: A warning of the dangers of social media. *Journal of Surgical Education, 71(6),* e28–32. doi:10.1016/j.jsurg.2014.05.013

Lunden, I. (2013, December 30). 73% of US adults use social networks, Pinterest passes Twitter in popularity, Facebook stays on top. Retrieved from http://techcrunch.com/2013/12/30/pew-social-networking/

MacDonald, J., Sohn, S., & Ellis, P. (2010). Privacy, professionalism and Facebook: A dilemma for young doctors. *Medical Education, 44*(8), 805–813. doi:10.1111/j.1365-2923.2010.03720.x

Moubarak, G., Guiot, A., Benhamou, Y., Benhamou, A., & Hariri, S. (2011). Facebook activity of residents and fellows and its impact on the doctor-patient relationship. *Journal of Medical Ethics, 37*(2), 101–104. doi:10.1136/jme.2010.036293

Osman, A., Wardle, A., & Caesar, R. (2012). Online professionalism and Facebook—falling through the generation gap. *Medical Teacher, 34*(8), e549–556. doi:10.3109/0142159X.2012.668624

Patel, P.D., Roberts, J.L., Miller, K.H., Ziegler, C., & Ostapchuk, M. (2012). The responsible use of online social networking: Who should mentor medical students. *Teaching and Learning in Medicine, 24*(4), 348–354. doi:10.1080/10401334.2012.715260

Ponce, B.A., Determann, J.R., Boohaker, H.A., Sheppard, E., McGwin, G., & Theiss, S. (2013). Social networking profiles and professionalism issues in residency applicants: An original study-cohort study. *Journal of Surgical Education, 70*(4), 502–507. doi:10.1016/j.jsurg.2013.02.005

Rocha, P.N., & de Castro, N.A.A. (2014). Opinions of students from a Brazilian medical school regarding online professionalism. *Journal of General Internal Medicine, 29*(5), 758–764. doi:10.1007/s11606-013-2748-y

Ross, S., Lai, K., Walton, J.M., Kirwan, P., & White, J.S. (2013). 'I have the right to a private life': Medical students' views about professionalism in a digital world. *Medical Teacher, 35*(10), 826–831. doi:10.3109/0142159X.2013.802301

Shore, R., Halsey, J., Shah, K., Crigger, B.-J., Douglas, S.P., & AMA Council on Ethical and Judicial Affairs. (2011). Report of the AMA Council on Ethical and Judicial Affairs: Professionalism in the use of social media. *Journal of Clinical Ethics, 22*(2), 165–172.

Thompson, L.A., Black, E., Duff, W.P., Paradise Black, N., Saliba, H., & Dawson, K. (2011). Protected health information on social networking sites: Ethical and legal considerations. *Journal of Medical Internet Research, 13*, e8. doi:10.2196/jmir.1590

Thompson, L.A., Dawson, K., Ferdig, R., Black, E.W., Boyer, J., Coutts, J., & Black, N.P. (2008). The intersection of online social networking with medical professionalism. *Journal of General Internal Medicine, 23*(7), 954–957. doi:10.1007/s11606-008-0538-8

White, J., Kirwan, P., Lai, K., Walton, J., & Ross, S. (2013). 'Have you seen what is on Facebook?' The use of social networking software by healthcare professions students. *BMJ Open, 3*(7), e003013. doi:10.1136/bmjopen-2013-003013.

Online social support networks

NEIL MEHTA[1] & ASHISH ATREJA[2]

[1]Cleveland Clinic, Lerner College of Medicine, Case Western Reserve University, Cleveland, Ohio, and
[2]Icahn School of Medicine at Mount Sinai, New York, USA

Abstract

Peer support groups have a long history and have been shown to improve health outcomes. With the increasing familiarity with online social networks like Facebook and ubiquitous access to the Internet, online social support networks are becoming popular. While studies have shown the benefit of these networks in providing emotional support or meeting informational needs, robust data on improving outcomes such as a decrease in health services utilization or reduction in adverse outcomes is lacking. These networks also pose unique challenges in the areas of patient privacy, funding models, quality of content, and research agendas. Addressing these concerns while creating patient-centred, patient-powered online support networks will help leverage these platforms to complement traditional healthcare delivery models in the current environment of value-based care.

Online social networking for patients

Peer support has been defined as social emotional support, frequently coupled with instrumental support, that is mutually offered or provided by individuals having a mental health condition to others sharing a similar condition to bring about a desired social or personal change (Gartner & Riessman, 1982). Peer support and self-help groups have long been popular among patients with mental health problems and other chronic and serious conditions. With the popularity of the Internet and increasingly ubiquitous access to it, there has been increasing interest in leveraging this technology to create virtual communities for patients. In this paper we will look at the evidence regarding the effectiveness of these social networking communities for providing support to patients and the challenges they face. We will conclude with recommendations for an ideal patient-centred online social network.

The practice of peer support in psychiatry has been traced back to 18th-century France when a hospital in Paris hired former patients to provide care to the sick. This was done as former patients were felt to be more gentle, honest and humane (Weiner, 1979). In the 1920s patients who had recovered from psychotic episodes were employed in inpatient units in the USA (Davidson et al., 2012). There have been many studies of the use of peer support for mental health conditions. Initially these studies showed that it was feasible and safe to use non-professional personnel to provide healthcare. Subsequent studies showed that peers could provide care comparable to professionals and could improve outcomes in specific areas like reduction in utilization of emergency rooms and hospitals, improved engagement of difficult to reach patients and some benefits in cases of substance abuse (Davidson et al., 2012; Rowe et al., 2007). The success demonstrated by these earlier studies prompted studies of the unique benefits that the experience and empathy of former patients can bring to the care of current patients (Davidson et al., 2012).

Self-help groups are the oldest and most pervasive of peer support types (Solomon, 2004). With the growth of the Internet, online support groups have come into existence. These groups lack the face-to-face element of the traditional self-help groups and thus add an element of anonymity, ease of access and openness (Davison et al., 2000; Perron, 2002).

The initial online support groups used asynchronous communication tools such as e-mails and bulletin boards with specific software such as Internet Relay Chat (IRC) for live communications. These tools allow for convenience and continuity while leveraging a larger support network.

We have come a long way from the early days of the Internet. With the popularity of the World Wide Web (web), it is often the first place a person turns to when faced with a new medical problem.

The journey may start with a Google search which can result in an overwhelming amount of information and can lead a person to ask for help in a social network either online or offline (Pang et al., 2014; Sarasohn-Kahn, 2008). The Internet is thus rivalling the physician as a source of health information. In fact, this online information-seeking behaviour is often prompted by a visit to a physician which may be unsatisfying and cause increased worry, disappointment, curiosity or loss of trust (Bell et al., 2011). In the USA 70–80% of all adult Internet users seek health information online, as it is often free, convenient, and has a wealth of information that patients can pursue at their own pace (Monteith et al., 2013). Of all those who use the Internet, 25–30% participate in online support groups related to medical conditions and personal problems (Fallows, 2005). As the healthcare system is burdened by an ageing population with multiple chronic problems, it is time to consider the use of online peer support groups to help better manage these problems.

What are the characteristics of an online support group?

Online support groups are somewhat like an online community of practice, where participants have a shared goal and desire to help and support each other. Being online, users can be geographically and temporally separated. The participants have mutual trust and a sense of anonymity and thus feel more able to talk about sensitive issues (Dosani et al., 2014). In addition there may be the ability to share multimedia (e.g. videos) and communicate via synchronous channels.

Is there evidence that these online support groups work?

Most of the research regarding the use of online support groups has been done in the context of specific conditions such as substance abuse (Rowe et al., 2007) or depression (Rice et al., 2014), or non-mental health conditions such as irritable bowel syndrome (Coulson, 2005) or cancer (Hong et al., 2012). Most of these studies are not high-quality randomized control trials; for example one systematic review of the use of Internet support groups for treatment of depression selected 28 trials for review and found that only 10 involved a randomized controlled trial (RCT)(Griffiths et al., 2009). Another systematic review of the outcomes of online support for cancer survivors found 37 articles that satisfied inclusion criteria and of these only four studies employed a RCT design (Hong et al., 2012). The outcomes measured showed some positive psychosocial effects but not in the RCTs.

Regardless of this lack of high-quality studies and hard outcomes, numerous studies have shown the benefits of online support groups. Users find online social networks helpful and more informative than static information web sites, they find it easier to talk to strangers than to family and friends and to communicate online rather than on a telephone (Jones et al., 2011). In one study patients with bipolar disorders found social networking to be very important for sharing emotions and to discuss their daily struggles with illness (Bauer et al., 2012). A survey of patients using cancer-related discussion groups provides support for a model that this social interaction led to increased social support and positive health outcomes in terms of depression, coping and stress (Beaudoin & Tao, 2007). Another survey of current users of online social networks revealed that users have two primary needs, emotional support and information- seeking, and they find different ways to use the networks to satisfy these needs. Those seeking emotional support tend to use more 'friending' and sharing of personal stories, while those seeking information tend to limit their use to discussion boards (Chung, 2014). Providing support can also have beneficial effects. A study of 114 pregnant members of eight pregnancy-related social networking sites did not show any health-related outcomes but did indicate that providing support was associated with seeking more information and following recommendations (Hether et al., 2014). A thematic analysis of 572 messages posted in a support group for individuals for irritable bowel syndrome revealed five categories of social support – emotional, esteem, information, network, and tangible assistance. In this group, informational support was the primary need with focus on areas of symptom interpretation, management and advice regarding interaction with healthcare professionals (Coulson, 2005). As may be expected, these needs may vary by the disease condition. A similar thematic analysis of an online discussion forum for patients with alcoholism found that the main categories of posts were 'sharing', 'supporting' and 'sobriety' supporting the role of the forum for practical and emotional benefit to users (Coulson, 2013).

These advantages, paired with the popularity of and easy access to online social networks, have led to a proliferation of online support groups. An indicator of the importance of such online networks is the funding by the Patient-Centered Outcomes Research Institute (PCORI) of 'patient-powered research networks' (PPRNs). These networks are operated and governed by groups of patients and their partners who are focused on a particular condition and interested in sharing health information and participating in research (PCORI, 2013).

Online support groups can be classified into two main categories.

1. Popular social networks (e.g. Facebook)
2. Healthcare-specific online support networks

    a. Networks addressing multiple or any health condition (e.g. PatientsLikeMe, DailyStrength)
    b. Condition-specific online support networks (e.g. Alzconnected, Mood PPRN (Nierenberg, 2013))

Popular social networks

While there are many popular social networks like Facebook, Google+ and Twitter there is most data for the use of Facebook for social support. Facebook is the largest online social network with over 1.3 billion members all over the world (Statista, 2014). Since almost everyone who has access to the Internet either via a desktop, laptop or mobile device has a Facebook account, it has become the default tool for staying in touch with friends and family. Thus people faced with a new medical problem can turn there for support much like they would reach out to a close contact in real life. Most popular social networking sites like Facebook or Google+ have an embedded instant message tool and an indicator if a 'friend' is online. Having a friend available online to communicate via instant messaging has been shown to be beneficial; it improves self-efficacy, decrease in stress and increased likelihood of seeking support (Feng & Hyun, 2012). The ease of use and access to these networks make them a tempting platform to use when seeking support. The user does not need to search for an appropriate group, create another account and learn how to navigate a new site or become familiar with its etiquette or customs. Thus a person faced with a new medical challenge can post a status update with a direct or implied cry for help. This could provide some benefit in the form of emotion sharing. Depending on the number of 'friends' and the prevalence of the medical problem, the user may be able to connect with another person who might be able to provide peer support and also meet the information needs and provide empathy.

This use of a popular social network for support does raise concerns. Firstly, such a post and response can reveal a user's personal medical history to all his 'friends'. While Google+ was designed from the ground up to limit unintentional sharing, the process of limiting the audience of a post is less obvious on Facebook. Most users on Facebook make their posts visible to all their contacts, including casual acquaintances and colleagues and 'bosses' at work. Secondly, the chances of finding a peer for a comparatively uncommon condition within one's circle of friends on a social network is unlikely.

Thirdly, both these factors would mean a person seeking emotional support may get no response or only very superficial unhelpful responses to their cry for help. This has the potential for adverse consequences on a person's mental health when he is the most vulnerable.

Fourthly, there is evidence that participation on such popular social networks may actually have negative effects, causing depression and jealousy (Kross et al., 2013). This is not unexpected as these networks have become optimal sites for practising impression management. When a person posts to an audience of people he knows in real-life, it difficult not to imagine what impression the post will create and how it will contribute to the poster's persona (Schlenker, 1980). This leads to posts of travels to exotic locations, fabulous dinners and selfies with celebrities. When the culture of a network is so different from the intention of a user seeking emotional support, it may be quite optimistic to expect such a platform to provide an ideal milieu for a person with a serious and sensitive mental health condition.

Aside from posting to the open stream or timeline, online social networks also allow for communities or groups with various levels of privacy. Users can find such groups by searching on the social network and join without needing to create a new user account. This creates a low bar for entry and can put the user in touch with peers whom they do not know from real life. There is no easy way to verify that a particular user really has a particular condition. Achieving a balance between privacy and openness is difficult to achieve. Thus a group of self-identified users with a particular health problem on a popular social network sets itself up to be targeted by other users with ulterior motives. A study of 15 diabetes support groups on Facebook, for example, found that 1/3 of the posts were for non-FDA approved remedies (Greene et al., 2011). To compound the problem, social networks have been encouraging users to use their real names and create authentic profiles. This prevents users from being anonymous even in private groups and thus excludes the biggest potential benefit of a peer support group. Even though it is possible to protect one's private information while being a member of a support group within a social network, the settings can be confusing and a user is one mouse click away for inadvertently exposing his sensitive information to a large group of strangers. The risk of such disclosure probably negates the potential benefit of the low bar to entry of a familiar network. Facebook has recently started working on leveraging its position as a leader of social networking to create online support communities with anonymity of users. While this sounds like a step in the right direction, the concern will be how much will the company itself learn about the users even if they are anonymous from each other (Farr & Oreskovic, 2014). Recently Facebook conducted an experiment on users by modifying their news feed to study the impact on their mood without their express consent (Kramer et al., 2014). Such lack of sensitivity limits severely the potential for healthy social support groups on a platform hosted by publicly traded companies that may not have their users' best interest at heart.

Healthcare-specific online social networks

Online social networks can be dedicated to specific health conditions such as substance abuse, or be broadly organized around multiple or any health-related condition. Use of these networks requires creation of an independent account which allows for anonymity and permits open discussion of sensitive topics. There is less risk of inadvertent disclosure of sensitive information. Since the company hosting the network does not know personal information about a user or his or her friends, there is less risk of loss of privacy. The concentration of other users with similar problems ensures an empathetic and helpful response. It is likely that except for patients with a single uncommon condition, a network that covers multiple common problems might be ideal for most

users. Since a number of chronic conditions have associated problems, it might be better to be on networks that have user groups that cover all these in one place. Thus a person with anxiety disorder may also have a history of substance abuse. It may be optimal for the person to be able to find peers with each problem and potentially start a subgroup of people with both problems.

The Internet is typically discussed as if it were a set of activities when it is actually a medium upon which various activities can occur. It is, therefore, neither 'good' nor 'bad' for mental health, although specific activities may have more influence than others (Bell, 2007). While many healthcare-specific support networks hold potential for benefit there is also a concern regarding the growth of online negative enabling support groups (ONESG) or 'extreme communities' which encourage negative or harmful behaviours (Haas et al., 2010). Typical examples of these are the 'pro-ana' websites that provide specific instructions for initiating and maintaining anorexia nervosa. These can be more numerous and better organized than sites maintained by professional services or those intended to support recovery (Chesley et al., 2003). Similarly, other extreme communities such as 'pro-suicide' and 'pro-amputation' groups can be found online (Bell, 2007). It is essential for

Table 1. Features of an ideal online social support network.

Ideal features	Comments
Patient-centred, patient-powered	The network must meet the needs of the patient; the best way to achieve this is to have patients manage it
No conflict of interest	The good of the patient must have the highest priority in any financial or research decisions. The decisions must involve patients and be fully transparent
Goal directed	The aim of the social network should be explicitly mentioned (e.g. support group for a disease, health communication between care providers and patients)
Trusted or moderated content	Some degree of moderation by healthcare personnel or a trusted organization would enhance credibility of information shared in social networks
Ability to remain anonymous	While HIPAA laws are not applicable if patients decide to release any information about themselves, networks must allow patients full control over anonymity and privacy
Intuitive user-interface	Networks should have intuitive user interfaces and user experiences to help ease adoption by patients at different levels of computer skills
Synchronous communication option	The platform should have a secure synchronous communication option, e.g. online chat, teleconference or video call, that allows patients to connect to each other in real time and get peer-counselling
Mobile access	The network should be accessible any time, any place across various devices (e.g. smartphones, tablets, desktop computers)
Gathering structured data	The platform should support tools or widgets to capture structured data through surveys or web form and should allow for risk stratification and support data visualization for feedback
Sharing data	Tools or widgets that allow sharing of structured data (such as from wearable devices, web forms) and unstructured data (such as web links, discussions)
Guidance for high-risk patients	As patient-powered social networks evolve, they should develop policies/procedures to screen and guide high-risk patients. These policies become essential in networks moderated by care providers. Additionally, there should be built-in tools to trigger proactive contact/support when there is an urgent risk identified
Outcome measurement	The platform should be designed (with patient consent) to collect data that would support research into the effectiveness in improving health outcomes. This evidence will support future funding of such networks and inform care providers when referring patients

HIPAA, US Health Insurance Portability and Accountability Act, 1996.

healthcare professionals to be aware of these ONESGs when treating vulnerable patients who are often stigmatized by their conditions and crave support.

One of the best new models of support groups is the PCORI funded PPRNs (PCORI, 2013), an example being the mood PPRN for patients with depression and bipolar disorder (Nierenberg, 2013). Since these are funded by a non-commercial entity and run by patients, the risk of loss of privacy is much less. These communities also drive the research agenda with the mood PPRN being centred on patients as collaborators to form a new patient–researcher–clinician community. The community captures patient-reported outcomes to conduct comparative effectiveness trials which will advance understanding of the biology of mood disorders for personalized care (Nierenberg, 2013).

Regardless of benefits, patients using the web for health information face challenges of variability in the quality of content, privacy issues and consumer fraud that are compounded by their own lack of technical skills and search competence (Monteith et al., 2013). In addition, users can come across inappropriate posts that can trigger traumatic memories, or hateful or abusive comments (flaming), and thus it is important for support groups to have moderators who can monitor the discussions. The moderators can also watch out for posts signalling potentially dangerous behaviours and act accordingly (Dosani et al., 2014). It is important to get health professionals to participate in such support networks, but a national survey revealed that physicians have concerns regarding ethics and confidentiality and are generally pessimistic regarding the role of online social networks (Bosslet et al., 2011).

The ideal online social support network would achieve the right balance between flexibility and security, anonymity and authenticity, openness and moderation, and be patient-centred and patient-powered while encouraging appropriate participation by healthcare providers (Table 1). The PPRNs are a step in the right direction and with the research agenda can help provide evidence for positive health outcomes.

Conclusions

As more users become familiar with social networks and Internet access becomes more ubiquitous, online social support groups have the potential to improve outcomes in an environment of value-based care. While a number of studies show benefits of such support groups, more robust research is need to study the impact on 'hard' outcomes. Such data will encourage healthcare providers to recommend appropriate support groups to their patients and even participate

in them. Care must be taken to develop the right financial and social model to protect the patient and leverage the technology to enhance patient centred research.

Declaration of interest: The authors report no conflicts of interest. The authors alone are responsible for the content and writing of the paper.

References

Bauer, R., Bauer, M., Spiessl, H., & Kagerbauer, T. (2012). Cyber-support: An analysis of online self-help forums (online self-help forums in bipolar disorder). *Nordic Journal of Psychiatry*, *67*(3), 185–190. doi:10.3109/08039488.2012.700734

Beaudoin, C.E., & Tao, C.-C. (2007). Benefiting from social capital in online support groups: An empirical study of cancer patients. *CyberPsychology and Behavior*, *10*(4), 587–590. doi:10.1089/cpb.2007.9986

Bell, R.A., Hu, X., Orrange, S.E., & Kravitz, R.L. (2011). Lingering questions and doubts: Online information-seeking of support forum members following their medical visits. *Patient Education and Counseling*, *85*(3), 525–528. doi:10.1016/j.pec.2011.01.015

Bell, V. (2007). Online information, extreme communities and Internet therapy: Is the Internet good for our mental health? *Journal of Mental Health*, *16*(4), 445–457. doi:10.1080/09638230701482378

Bosslet, G., Torke, A., Hickman, S., Terry, C., & Helft, P. (2011). The patient–doctor relationship and online social networks: Results of a national survey. *Journal of General Internal Medicine*, *26*(10), 1168–1174. doi:10.1007/s11606-011-1761-2

Chesley, E.B., Alberts, J.D., Klein, J.D., & Kreipe, R.E. (2003). Pro or con? Anorexia nervosa and the Internet. *Journal of Adolescent Health*, *32*(2), 123–124. doi:10.1016/S1054-139X(02)00615-8

Chung, J.E. (2014). Social networking in online support groups for health: How online social networking benefits patients. *Journal of Health Communication*, *19*(6), 639–659. doi:10.1080/10810730.2012.757396

Coulson, N.S. (2005). Receiving social support online: An analysis of a computer-mediated support group for individuals living with irritable bowel syndrome. *CyberPsychology and Behavior*, *8*(6), 580–584. doi:10.1089/cpb.2005.8.580

Coulson, N.S. (2013). Sharing, supporting and sobriety: A qualitative analysis of messages posted to alcohol-related online discussion forums in the United Kingdom. *Journal of Substance Use*, *19*(1–2), 176–180. doi:10.3109/14659891.2013.765516

Davidson, L., Bellamy, C., Guy, K., & Miller, R. (2012). Peer support among persons with severe mental illnesses: A review of evidence and experience. *World Psychiatry*, *11*(2), 123–128.

Davison, K.P., Pennebaker, J.W., & Dickerson, S.S. (2000). Who talks? The social psychology of illness support groups. *American Psychologist*, *55*(2), 205–217.

Dosani, S., Harding, C., & Wilson, S. (2014). Online groups and patient forums. *Current Psychiatry Reports*, *16*(11), 507. doi:10.1007/s11920-014-0507-3

Fallows, D. (2005). Part 5. Functions of the Internet: How men and women use it as a tool to communicate, transact, get information, and entertain themselves. Washington, DC: Pew Research Center. Retrieved from http://www.pewinternet.org/2005/12/28/part-5-functions-of-the-internet-how-men-and-women-use-it-as-a-tool-to-communicate-transact-get-information-and-entertain-themselves/

Farr, C., & Oreskovic, A. (2014, October 3). Exclusive: Facebook plots first steps into healthcare. San Francisco: Reuters. Retrieved from http://www.reuters.com/article/2014/10/03/us-facebook-health-idUSKCN0HS09720141003

Feng, B., & Hyun, M.J. (2012). The influence of friends' instant messenger status on individuals' coping and support-seeking. *Communication Studies, 63*(5), 536–553. doi:10.1080/10510974.2011.649443

Gartner, A.J., & Riessman, F. (1982). Self-help and mental health. *Hospital and Community Psychiatry, 33*(8), 631–635.

Greene, J.A., Choudhry, N.K., Kilabuk, E., & Shrank, W.H. (2011). Online social networking by patients with diabetes: A qualitative evaluation of communication with Facebook. *Journal of General Internal Medicine, 26*(3), 287–292. doi:10.1007/s11606-010-1526-3

Griffiths, K.M., Calear, A.L., & Banfield, M. (2009). Systematic review on Internet support groups (ISGs) and depression (1): Do ISGs reduce depressive symptoms? *Journal of Medical Internet Research, 11*(3), e40. doi:10.2196/jmir.1270

Haas, S.M., Irr, M.E., Jennings, N.A., & Wagner, L.M. (2010). Online negative enabling support groups. *New Media and Society,* 1461444810363910. doi:10.1177/1461444810363910

Hether, H.J., Murphy, S.T., & Valente, T.W. (2014). It's better to give than to receive: The role of social support, trust, and participation on health-related social networking sites. *Journal of Health Communication, 19*(12), 1424–1439. doi:10.1080/10810730.2014.894596

Hong, Y., Peña-Purcell, N.C., & Ory, M.G. (2012). Outcomes of online support and resources for cancer survivors: A systematic literature review. *Patient Education and Counseling, 86*(3), 288–296. doi:10.1016/j.pec.2011.06.014

Jones, R., Sharkey, S., Ford, T., Emmens, T., Hewis, E., Smithson, J., ... Owens, C. (2011). Online discussion forums for young people who self-harm: User views. *Psychiatrist, 35*(10), 364–368. doi:10.1192/pb.bp.110.033449

Kramer, A.D.I., Guillory, J.E., & Hancock, J.T. (2014). Experimental evidence of massive-scale emotional contagion through social networks. *Proceedings of the National Academy of Sciences, 111*(24), 8788–8790. doi:10.1073/pnas.1320040111

Kross, E., Verduyn, P., Demiralp, E., Park, J., Lee, D.S., Lin, N., ... Ybarra, O. (2013). Facebook use predicts declines in subjective well-being in young adults. *PLoS ONE, 8*(8), e69841. doi:10.1371/journal.pone.0069841

Monteith, S., Glenn, T., & Bauer, M. (2013). Searching the Internet for health information about bipolar disorder: Some cautionary issues. *International Journal of Bipolar Disorders, 1*(1), 22. doi:10.1186/2194-7511-1-22

Nierenberg, A.A. (2013). Mood Patient-Powered Research Network. PCORI. Retrieved from http://www.pcori.org/node/4403

Pang, P., Chang, S., Pearce, J., & Verspoor, K. (2014). Online health information seeking behaviour: Understanding different search approaches. *PACIS Proceedings, 2014, 229.* Retrieved from http://aisel.aisnet.org/pacis2014/229

PCORI. (2013). Clinical data and patient-powered research networks: Awarded projects. Patient-Centered Outcomes Research Institute. Retrieved from http://www.pcori.org/content/clinical-data-and-patient-powered-research-networks-awarded-projects

Perron, B. (2002). Online support for caregivers of people with a mental illness. *Psychiatric Rehabilitation Journal, 26,* 70–77.

Rice, S.M., Goodall, J., Hetrick, S.E., Parker, A.G., Gilbertson, T., Amminger, G.P., ... Alvarez-Jimenez, M. (2014). Online and social networking interventions for the treatment of depression in young people: A systematic review. *Journal of Medical Internet Research, 16*(9), e206. doi:10.2196/jmir.3304

Rowe, M., Bellamy, C., Baranoski, M., Wieland, M., O'Connell, M.J., Benedict, P., ... Sells, D. (2007). A peer-support, group intervention to reduce substance use and criminality among persons with severe mental illness. *Psychiatric Services, 58*(7), 955–961. doi:10.1176/appi.ps.58.7.955

Sarasohn-Kahn, J. (2008). The wisdom of patients: Health care meets online social media. Caliornia Health Care Foundation. Retrieved from http://www.chcf.org/publications/2008/04/the-wisdom-of-patients-health-care-meets-online-social-media

Schlenker, B.R. (1980). *Impression Management: The Self-Concept, Social Identity, and Interpersonal Relations.* Monterey, CA: Brooks/Cole.

Solomon, P. (2004). Peer support/peer provided services underlying processes, benefits, and critical ingredients. *Psychiatric Rehabilitation Journal, 27*(4), 392–401.

Statista. (2014). Number of monthly active Facebook users 2008–2014. Retrieved 16 October 2014 from http://www.statista.com/statistics/264810/number-of-monthly-active-facebook-users-worldwide/

Weiner, D.B. (1979). The apprenticeship of Philippe Pinel: A new document, 'Observations of Citizen Pussin on the insane.' *American Journal of Psychiatry, 136*(9), 1128–1134.

Social media for lifelong learning

TERRY KIND[1] & YOLANDA EVANS[2]

[1]*Children's National Health System, George Washington University School of Medicine, Washington DC, USA,* *and* [2]*Seattle Children's Hospital, University of Washington, Seattle, Washington, USA,*

Abstract

Learning is ongoing, and can be considered a social activity. In this paper we aim to provide a review of the use of social media for lifelong learning. We start by defining lifelong learning, drawing upon principles of continuous professional development and adult learning theory. We searched Embase and MEDLINE from 2004–2014 for search terms relevant to social media and learning. We describe examples of lifelong learners using social media in medical education and healthcare that have been reported in the peer-reviewed literature. Medical or other health professions students may have qualities consistent with being a lifelong learner, yet once individuals move beyond structured learning environments they will need to recognize their own gaps in knowledge and skills over time and be motivated to fill them, thereby incorporating lifelong learning principles into their day-to-day practice. Engagement with social media can parallel engagement in the learning process over time, to the extent that online social networking fosters feedback and collaboration. The use of social media and online networking platforms are a key way to continuously learn in today's information sharing society. Additional research is needed, particularly rigorous studies that extend beyond learner satisfaction to knowledge, behaviour change, and outcomes.

Introduction

Do we ever stop learning? And is there anyone from whom we cannot learn something? To the extent that learning is social and ongoing, then even as adults, humans continue to interact and learn. Learning has been considered a social activity by psychologists such as Albert Bandura, who theorized that we learn by modelling others, and Lev Vygotsky, who proposed that we learn through social interaction (Taylor & Hamdy, 2013; Yardley et al., 2012). Some of our interactions are collaborative, others competitive; some are among peer groups, others are hierarchical; some occur in real time, and others by taking turns. Increasingly, our interactions may be widely spaced geographically, and among people who do not otherwise know each other except through a common topic of interest about which learning and sharing occurs. One technological enhancement to facilitate these processes is online social networking.

Social networking site use has increased among all age groups over time; 89% of young adult American Internet users and more than two thirds of American Internet users age 30–64 use social networking sites (Pew Research Center, 2014). Even among senior American adult Internet users over the age of 65, almost half (46%) are using social networking (Pew Research Center, 2014). Social media can be thought of as the content shared on such sites, and is a term often used interchangeably with social networking.

In this article we aim to provide a review of the use of social media for lifelong learning. We start by defining lifelong learning itself, and in doing so we describe the theoretical underpinnings of the adult learner. We explore the conditions under which lifelong learning occurs. This sets the context for our search for various examples reported in the peer-reviewed literature of how social media is used by lifelong learners, drawing upon principles of continuous professional development and adult learning theory. Examples span a range from video platforms to microblogs and are at times multidisciplinary and across fields; each has applicability to lifelong learning.

Search strategy

For this review, we sought to identify reports of social media use for lifelong learning that have been reported in the peer-reviewed literature. We searched EMBASE and Medline from 2004–2014 using the following search terms: medical education, continuing medical education, graduate medical education, undergraduate medical education, internship, residency, lifelong learning, blogging, social media, Twitter, Facebook, online journal club. We also included relevant citations identified from the reference lists of the articles retrieved.

What is lifelong learning?

Definitions

Taken literally, lifelong learners are those people who continue to learn over time. Broadly defined, lifelong learning is the development of human potential in the areas of knowledge, values and skills, through a continuously supportive process that is stimulating and empowering and that fosters confidence, creativity, and enjoyment in all roles and circumstances (Hojat et al., 2003). This is difficult to operationalize, but there have been several studies which have aimed to do just that. As an example, in developing the Jefferson Lifelong Learning Scale among physicians, Hojat et al. (2003, 2009) identified the following underlying factors of lifelong learning: (1) recognition of one's own learning needs, (2) participation in research endeavours, (3) self-initiation or self-directed learning, (4) technical/computer skills, and (5) personal motivation. Among medical students, the key concepts identified that pertained to their lifelong learning were their learning beliefs and motivation, their skills in seeking information, and their attention to learning opportunities (Wetzel et al., 2010).

Lifelong learning continues beyond formal instructional periods throughout one's life, and has also been called career-long learning (Burman et al., 2014). Depending on the nature of one's career, this may be framed as staff/faculty development, professional development, continuing education, continuous professional development or any number of other related terms. In any case, it is reasonably accepted that lifelong learning will be most effective when self-directed and applicable to the motivated adult learner.

Who is the adult learner? What do the theories of adult learning say?

In identifying the characteristic features of adults who are going to continue to learn over time, we can draw upon various adult learning theories. Self-directed adult learners have been classically described by Malcolm Knowles (2005) as internally motivated and drawing upon their prior experience to aid in their learning. They are responsible for and involved in planning their learning based on their need to know something and their drive to apply what they have learned immediately. What they learn is related to their role in society.

Merriam and Caffarella (1999) also note that the learning that goes on in adulthood is shaped by socio-cultural context and can be understood through examining the social context in which it occurs. What one learns, what opportunities are available, and the manner in which one learns are largely determined by the society in which one lives (Merriam & Caffarella, 1999). Here and now, in this digital age, there is an online society with increasing opportunities for learning within and across online networks over time, which forms the basis for this paper.

Other adult learning theories with potential applicability to lifelong learning in social networks that we will highlight include transformational, experiential, and social learning. Learning is transformational when the adult makes meaning of what they do (problem solving) and what they understand about others (communicative learning). Mezirow (1990) includes critical reflection as a component of transformational learning. Curricular content (what one learns) and educational processes (how one is taught) that support learners' critical reflection upon their own premises will foster transformational learning.

Kolb (1984) discusses experiential learning which is not achieved in a formal setting, but rather in the practice of reflection upon day-to-day experiences. Here, learning is 'making meaning' from real-life experiences which extend beyond the traditional workplace and beyond organized educational sessions. Experiential learning is consequential and can be maximized even when 'unstructured, unintended, and opportunistic' (Yardley et al., 2012, p. 163).

Social learning theory places an emphasis on communities of practice and the assumptions that learning and thinking are social activities, structured by the tools available in various learning situations (Taylor & Hamdy, 2013). Each of these theories of adult learning has relevance to current and future social media-based interactions, communities, and exchanges of ideas.

Why participate in lifelong learning, as a physician/healthcare professional?

One reason among many that physicians participate in lifelong learning is to stay current with the advances in their field. They may do this formally by maintaining accreditation with a certifying agency, such as participating in a Maintenance of Certification (MOC) programme. The American Board of Medical Specialties (ABMS) oversees the certification of physician specialists in 24 boards in the USA, and is charged with assuring (the public) that physicians participating in MOC are 'committed to lifelong learning and competency' in their speciality and/or subspeciality (ABMS, 2014). These physicians are demonstrating to the public that they are keeping up to date. Physicians participate in continuing education in part to satisfy licensing requirements; this involves practice-based learning and improvement, where they identify their gaps and then fill them, applying what they have learned directly in clinical practice. The process is formalized during residency training, where the US Accreditation Council for Graduate Medical Education (ACGME) holds that trainees should investigate and evaluate their clinical care, appraise and assimilate scientific evidence, and continuously 'improve patient care based on constant self-evaluation and lifelong learning' (ACGME, 2014).

Ultimately, it is part of medical professionalism and a physician's charter to be committed to self-directed lifelong learning (American Board of Internal Medicine et al., 2002). In addition, lifelong learning has been associated with career satisfaction, as found in a study of psychiatrists (Afonso et al., 2014). This suggests that the more physicians are motivated to stay current with developments in their field, the more satisfied they will be. In a rapidly changing field with vast amounts of new information, one might ask if social media can help foster the ongoing learning that it takes to stay up to date, as a lifelong learner, and perhaps foster career satisfaction along the way.

How does social media relate to lifelong learning?

Technology and social media have contributed to an information society, and can increase access to learning for people of all ages and potentially across socio-economic levels across the world (Merriam & Caffarella, 1999). Connecting through social media can bring those geographically diverse together in communication across time zones and continents. Hence, distance learning is an integral part of how social media relates to lifelong learning, as is any blended learning endeavour with networking and ongoing participation before or after a live session, for example.

Social media can extend real-life learning and relationships into a shared space to foster professional growth (Kind et al., 2013). Some of the key features of social media include its interactive nature, where information is shared either synchronously (in real time) and/or asynchronously through conversations, chats, comments, videos, and other interactions. The interactivity allows individual learners to share ideas, questions, and goals (with actual or virtual peers, faculty, mentors), and have accountability partners in the learning and practice improvement process. There is great potential for social media to break

down traditional hierarchies, for example, by providing medical students access to attending physicians, in the ongoing quest for knowledge and learning.

Engagement with social media can parallel engagement in the learning process to the extent that online social networking fosters feedback and collaboration. It can also provide a forum and format for reflection, through online blogging and other prompted discussions and journaling (Cheston et al., 2013). To be a reflective practitioner is part of professionalism, and to be a clinical educator is to foster lifelong learning in others (Schön, 1990).

With rapid easy access and ease of information-seeking and sharing, there is also online learning at the point of care, and other formal and informal opportunities to learn and share information. Reading blogged summaries with links to the peer-reviewed literature, participating in social media-based journal clubs, and classroom technology that links student to professor and other experts are becoming more common as social media becomes interdigitated with lifelong learning. Handheld technology and other portable computing options place social networking in the hands of physicians throughout their days and nights, and over a career where advancements are frequent and keeping up to date and communication with other experts in the field is critical.

In one study among physicians that aimed to identify the factors that influence physicians' use of social media as a component of their lifelong learning and continuing professional development, social media applications were seen as efficient and effective methods for keeping up to date and sharing newly acquired medical knowledge with others in the medical community (McGowan et al., 2012)

In this paper we look at the conditions that promote lifelong learning through examples of social media/networking reported in the peer-reviewed literature.

Which social media tools are being utilized for the promotion of lifelong learning?

With 74% of adults in the USA using social networking sites, there is ample opportunity to incorporate learning into this technology (Pew Research Center, 2014). There are numerous social media tools available for use. Each has unique advantages and disadvantages for the educator and learner. Tools that engage the learner include the use of an educator's perspective on a topic with opportunities for learner responses, questions, and contributions. Those that use video allow for visual demonstrations and typically incorporate audio as well, delivering visual and auditory (even auscultatory) content when, where, and how the learner is ready to learn. This section will provide examples of some of the main social media tools as they are used in various disciplines to enhance learning over time. For the purposes of this review we will focus on some examples of those that have been studied and published in peer reviewed literature.

Blogs

A web log, more commonly referred to as a blog, is an online log entry where the author(s) routinely update and maintain content or posts. Readers (at times, learners) can comment on the posts and authors (at times, educators) then respond in turn, asynchronously, resulting in a reciprocal read and response relationship between author and one or many readers. Blogging is commonly done by physicians to share opinions, health information, and updates on trending topics. It can be challenging for blog readers to differentiate fact from author opinion, and some medical blogs are used more as diaries than avenues for medical teaching. Despite these limitations, blogs have potential as learning tools. Individuals in medical school have used blogging to provide advice on preparation techniques for standardized tests, guidance on clinical rotations, and social support (Pinilla et al., 2013) and one institution has reported using blogging to engage residents in morning report (Bogoch et al., 2010). Journal club, the critical reading of peer reviewed articles to provide evidence-based practice guidelines in discussion format, has long been used in medical education. The use of a blog to promote and facilitate journal clubs ('live' and/or online 'virtual' journal clubs) has also been an effective way to engage healthcare providers (including trainees and students) and provide them with a resource that allows for efficient access to evidence-based medicine in an easy to search format (Genes & Parekh, 2010). Blogs often include hyperlinks to specific texts which allow for the reader to access information referenced in the blog post instantly, and if desired, allowing the reader (learner) to delve further into the subject in a self-directed manner. When blogging contains links to peer-reviewed evidence, for example when it is used for journal club, morning report, or in association with any teaching conference, the references are available to the reader to use over time (before, during, after a given 'live' session). This advantage makes blogs an ideal option for teaching evidence-based practice at the patient bedside, during rounds, and on an individual's own personal time. In addition, commenting functions allow for questions and answers, further reflections on the topic, and extension to additional topics that can inform future blog posts and additional learning.

Microblogs

Microblogs are similar to blogs, as they provide a shared space for posting information and receiving feedback. Their distinguishing feature is the brief nature of the posts, given that user comments and responses are limited to a certain character count, often 140 characters or less. While Twitter is the most commonly used microblog in the USA (Pew Research Center, 2014), there are numerous other microblog platforms available worldwide, varying in the degree to which they are used publicly or in closed groups. In dental education, the use of microblogs during classroom lectures has been shown to provide a more stimulating and engaging atmosphere for students (McAndrew & Johnston, 2012). Pharmacy students in China who were given the task of participating in group discussion using the popular microblog Sina Weibo, displayed improvements in participation and satisfaction with their course work. In this example, instructors tracked student participation on Sina Weibo. Over 80% of these students agreed that the microblog improved communication and the majority also agreed it increased their interaction in the course (Wang et al., 2013). In the USA, Twitter has been used to provide medical updates and clinical pearls about rheumatology topics to medical trainees and physicians (Collins, 2011). It was also a successful adjunct to a high yield ultrasonography curriculum. Students received daily 'tweets' over a year-long programme. Even students who had no prior experience with Twitter found the information useful and the platform user-friendly (Bahner et al., 2012). Twitter also has been used in conjunction with scientific and educational conferences, known as 'live tweeting', and addressed by Djuricich elsewhere in this journal's special social media edition.

Social media video feed

The use of lectures as well as hands-on bedside teaching has been the standard of medical education for centuries. Technology now allows for the option of video-based – including multi-media interactive – curricula to supplement and potentially enhance teaching in person. A common online site for sharing information via video feed is YouTube. Demonstrations of (and at times actual) procedures, such as knee arthrocentesis, are searchable and viewable, and shareable on YouTube. Though the educational quality is limited by the knowledge and skill of those creating and/or posting the videos, when they describe and take the learner clearly and systematically through a procedure, this can provide useful tips, recommendations, and early exposure to the procedure before it is taught in person and in real time (Fischer et al., 2013). Videos (of self or others) can also be available for review or possibly for remediation by learners after the demonstration, live performance, or in simulation. Other critical physical exam skills, such as cardiac and respiratory auscultation, have the potential to be taught with YouTube videos, but currently the quality of recordings is highly variable (Camm et al., 2013; Sunderland et al., 2014). Despite some limitations, YouTube has promising potential as a lifelong teaching tool when used for clinical education. Viewer comments can help with revision of video content and YouTube channels can be shared in a variety of online forums (blogs, microblogs, websites, and social networking sites) (Topps et al., 2013). Creation of a YouTube channel devoted to a specific health topic has been successful. Clinicians in North Carolina condensed 60-min nephrology lectures into 10-min videos and posted them on a YouTube channel. They asked healthcare providers their opinions on the videos. The majority of users considered the video format to be useful and over 80% of providers felt the information was accurate, current, and objective (Desai et al., 2013).

Collaborative writing applications

Collaborative writing applications (CWAs) include online document forums with the potential for multiple contributing authors who need not be in the same place or time. Examples include Google documents and wikis. These collaborative documents allow colleagues to continually update, edit, and add new information that is shared and easily accessible. An example of the potential for a wiki to improve patient care was described by Gupta et al. (2012). The purpose was to create an asthma action plan. They recruited providers from Canada, the USA and Australia to take part in working groups that would contribute to wikis. At the end of their study, nearly 75% of the participants were satisfied with the asthma action plan outcome (Gupta et al., 2012). A second example of lifelong learning using a CWA comes from the Medical College of Georgia's Physician Assistant Program (Lanning & Dadiq, 2010). In an effort to incorporate palliative care teaching, a wiki was built for students to document their experiences in adult medicine. Students who reported participating in the Wiki Discussion Forum reported a better understanding of end-of-life concerns. One review of CWAs found that much of the available literature on them is descriptive, such as observational case studies, and that while potential for learning and collaboration is high, contributions are relatively low (Archambault et al., 2013).

Social networking sites

Social networking sites such as Facebook are a common way of engaging users in social interactions.

Facebook currently has over 1 billion users worldwide, and other sites such as LinkedIn incorporate networking for professional career opportunities. These sites have the potential to enhance lifelong learning if used to support educational goals (such as study groups, or question/answer forums between students and educators). Social networking sites have been described in combination with other forms of social media (YouTube and Skype) to promote learning in continuing medical education (Wang et al., 2012). The use of a social network as the sole tool for supplementation of learning has been described in various educational settings. Bachelor of Nursing students in Queensland, Australia, were offered a study forum via Facebook to supplement a rigorous course during exam week. Participation in the group was voluntary with 70% of the student cohort joining. While their survey response rate was poor (24%), the authors describe that 92% of students found the group useful and inclusive (Tower, 2014). Facebook has been used in courses of anatomy, disease management, and pharmacology to enhance participation and promote discussion between educators and learners (DiVall & Kirwin, 2012; Estus, 2010; Jaffar, 2014).

Which social media tools work the best for the promotion of lifelong learning?

Traditional lifelong learning, in the form of educational seminars, conferences, or continuing medical education utilize a variety of formats for imparting knowledge and engaging the motivated learner to apply this knowledge to ongoing practice. These formats include, but are not limited to, small group activities, lectures, one-to-one teaching, workshops, journal clubs, and case-based conferences. Often a medical education conference will incorporate a variety of formats to impact a range of learners.

As with traditional lifelong learning, there is not one ideal method for education using social media tools. Learners will need information in a variety of formats, designed to fit the specific educational objectives, to fit different learning styles and preferences, and to fill the learner's gaps over time given new evidence, new opportunities, and new challenges. Methods of teaching that promote learner engagement are the most effective. Similarly, social media tools that engage the learner, provide accurate and up-to-date information, and can be easily modified to accommodate new and emerging research in specific subject areas are likely to be the most effective tools for lifelong learning. Educators at Penn State integrated the use of five social media tools into the fourth-year medical student curriculum in order to augment course work. They found that integrating social media in the classroom activities enhanced connection between the teacher and student, increased communication outside of the classroom, and led to more collaboration amongst students (George & Dellasega, 2011). In this example, the educators incorporated the use of social media in their formal teaching, but learners are likely seeking out multiple forms of online communication to enhance their own learning outside the formal setting. A survey of over 200 pre-medical students in the UK found that most students were using both instant messaging and social networking sites; even back in 2008, blogs were read by about 20% of the students and a fifth of the male students reported both using and contributing information to wikis (Sandars, 2008). With increasing use of these and similar interactive, collaborative, online tools and social media applications in the context of medical student education, more healthcare providers (upon graduation) will be at ease with and inclined to continue making use of social media for ongoing learning throughout their careers.

With this in mind, let us highlight social media tools that may be most beneficial for learning in specific settings. Also see Table 1 for opportunities and challenges.

In the classroom

Tools that encourage interaction, engagement, and collaboration, such as Facebook, Twitter, and blogs are innovative tools for the classroom, and as a stepping off point to extend learning beyond (pre/post) the classroom. In the examples listed previously, educators found that utilizing these social media

Table 1. Social media tools and opportunities and challenges for lifelong learning.

Social media tool	Opportunities for lifelong learning	Challenges for lifelong learning
Blog and microblog	Links to additional references Blog authors provide summarized perspectives and reactions to latest peer-reviewed research or to current events Allows for comments and questions by readership which can facilitate future content and enhancements Typically searchable for specific content Opportunities for learners/educators to identify knowledge gaps and create new posts to share with specific groups or publicly Subscribers (often for free) and followers receive updates and links to newly posted content Educator to learner (or learner to learner) reminders to complete educational "assignments" or answer queries Open access and widely available in multiple settings and via many devices Provides platform for reflections and opportunities for personal improvement Rapid, crowd-sourced answers to clinical questions; or "question of the week" with learners Provides or links to formal CME opportunities	Credibility of information varies Comments may be subject to moderation Many distractors from key learning questions Must actively avoid breaching patient confidentiality at all times
Video feed	"Traditional lectures" available and searchable by learners and can be viewed multiple times, can be viewed at rapid speed or slowed down; abbreviated/summary versions available Video demonstrations of procedures and physical exam techniques Opportunities for learners/educators to identify knowledge gaps and create new videos to post and share Learners can influence future content via commentary Potentially searchable for specific content Subscribers (often for free) and "channel" followers receive updates and links to newly posted content	Variable video quality Variable content quality (ex. procedures and exam techniques) Credibility of information varies Interactions with learners limited to commentary Must actively avoid breaching patient confidentiality
Wiki and collaborative writing applications (CWA)	Collaborative body of information updated by multiple authors Active contributions by learners with potential for feedback Content often includes links to peer-reviewed or other credible citations Content-specific wikis draw interest and contributions from experts and learners	Credibility of information varies Information can be overwritten Must actively avoid breaching patient confidentiality at all times

constructs led to increased learner participation as well as improved interaction with peers. There is also a potential to break down hierarchy and facilitate questions and answers among students, trainees, and faculty. Furthermore, with the use of social media, the live classroom can be either transformed into, or augmented by, a virtual one.

In clinical care

Tools that are readily accessible, provide easy access to peer-reviewed information, and can be revised based on user feedback and new developments are the most appropriate for settings such as the patient bedside, morning report, or journal clubs. These include the use of blogs and CWAs/wikis.

During the learner's personal time

All of the above forms of social media are accessible at any time of day or night; however, certain tools, such as video feed, may be most beneficial during the learner's own free time. Video feed allows the learner to see examples of procedures that may be of interest or hear portions of (or entire) traditional lectures at times that are convenient and at playback speeds of their choosing.

What are under-recognized tools for life-long learning?

There are many social networking sites and social media tools that are not currently found in the evidence-based literature. Examples include photo blogs such as Pinterest and Tumblr as well as social networking sites such as Reddit. While the popularity of such sites is constantly evolving, these media offer the unique advantage of being based mainly on visual images that then can link to other sites of information. On each of these platforms, the general public is posting information on health-related topics ranging from disease-specific supports to trends in weight management, nutrition, and behavioural health remedies. Healthcare professionals could make use of these to learn about trends in patient preferences and public perception of common and emerging health-related concerns.

What are some limitations/pitfalls?

We have showcased examples of how social media can be used for learning at the student, trainee, and medical professional level. The opportunities for enhancing traditional education and providing innovative ways to engage the learner throughout their careers, beyond the classroom, are important

advantages; however, there are limitations. At present, although there are guidelines for medical educators regarding standards of practice and tips to promote professionalism (Kind et al., 2013, 2014), rigorous evaluation of their effectiveness for teaching and learning are needed.

Social media tools afford opportunities, but the content is user-generated, often unverified by experts, and merely commented on by peers. The use of wikis and other collaborative online documents is an example of how content may or may not be monitored. Content may be inaccurate and contribution rates low.

As with any learning opportunity, and potentially to greater degree for social media, there is the possibility of drifting from the learning task. This could be a benefit if the learning is motivated by what is a pressing need or interest, or could be a hindrance if the learner is distracted.

Where are the gaps in the research on social media and lifelong learning?

The use of social media to augment learning is a relatively new and growing area. Additional research is needed, particularly studies that extend beyond learner satisfaction, to learner acquisition of knowledge, skills, attitudes, to behaviour change, and ultimately to patient care outcomes. There is also very little on the use of social networking sites to promote professional development; sites such as Doximity and LinkedIn have not been assessed in the peer-reviewed literature as tools for learning. Most, if not all of the studies published have been descriptive in nature rather than experimental. Appropriate comparison studies, and those rigorously assessing outcomes need to be conducted and disseminated. We anticipate the use of altmetrics (Priem et al., 2012) as contributing to the literature on social media for lifelong learning, particularly in terms of learner engagement.

Conclusions

Lifelong learning starts with learning itself. The medical or other health professions student who is currently in school can participate in lifelong learning, and have qualities consistent with being a lifelong learner. But it is once individuals are beyond structured learning environments that they will need to recognize their own knowledge and skills gaps over time and be motivated to fill them, and incorporate lifelong learning principles into their day-to-day practice. The use of social media and technology is one key way to do so, in today's information sharing society.

Declaration of interest: The authors report no conflicts of interest. The authors alone are responsible for the content and writing of the paper.

References

ABMS. (2014). About ABMS Maintenance of Certification. American Board of Medical Specialties. Retrieved from: http://www.abms.org/Maintenance_of_Certification/

ACGME. (2014). Accreditation Council for Graduate Medical Education. Retrieved from https://www.acgme.org/acgmeweb/

Afonso, P., Ramos, M.R., Saraiva, S., Moreira, C.A., & Figueira, M.L. (2014). Assessing the relation between career satisfaction in psychiatry with lifelong learning and scientific activity. *Psychiatry Research, 217,* 210–214.

American Board of Internal Medicine, American College of Physicians–American Society of Internal Medicine, European Federation of Internal Medicine. (2002). Medical professionalism in the new millennium: A physician charter. *Annals of Internal Medicine, 136,* 243–246.

Archambault, P.M., van de Belt, T.H., Grajales, F.J. III, Faber M.J., Kuziemsky, C.E., Gagnon, S., ... Légaré, F. (2013). Wikis and collaborative writing applications in health care: A scoping review. *Journal of Medical Internet Research, 15*(10), e210.

Bahner, D.P., Adkins, E., Patel, N., Donley, C., Nagel, R., & Kman, N.E. (2012). How we use social media to supplement a novel curriculum in medical education. *Medical Teacher, 34,* 439–444.

Bogoch, I.I., Frost, D.W., Bridge, S., Lee, T.C., Gold, W.L., Panisko, D.M., & Cavalcanti, R.B. (2010). Morning report blog: A web-based tool to enhance case-based learning. *Teaching & Learning in Medicine, 24,* 238–241.

Burman, N.J., Boscardin, C.K., Van Schaik, S.M. (2014). Career-long learning: Relationship between cognitive and metacognitive skills. *Medical Teacher, 36,* 715–723.

Camm, C.F., Sunderland, N., & Camm, A.J. (2013). A quality assessment of cardiac auscultation material on YouTube. *Clinical Cardiology, 36,* 77–81.

Cheston, C.C., Flickinger, T.E., & Chisolm, M.S. (2013). Social media use in medical education: A systematic review. *Academic Medicine, 88,* 893–901.

Collins, C.E. (2011). Twitter and rheumatology based medical education analysis of the first 100 followers. *Arthritis and Rheumatism, 63*(10), S29.

Desai, T., Sanghani, V., Fang, X., Christiano, C., & Ferris, M. (2013). Assessing a nephrology-focused YouTube channel's potential to educate health care providers. *Journal of Nephrology, 26,* 81–85.

DiVall, M.V., & Kirwin, J.L. (2012). Using Facebook to facilitate course-related discussion between students and faculty members. *American Journal of Pharmaceutical Education, 76, 2,* 32.

Estus, E.L. (2010). Using facebook within a geriatric pharmacotherapy course. *American Journal of Pharmaceutical Education, 74,* 145–149.

Fischer, J., Geurts, J., Valderrabano, V., & Hügle, T. (2013). Educational quality of YouTube videos on knee arthrocentesis. *Journal of Clinical Rheumatology, 19,* 373–376.

Genes, N., Parekh, S. (2010). Bringing journal club to the bedside in the form of a critical appraisal blog. *Journal of Emergency Medicine, 39,* 504–505.

George, D.R, & Dellasega, C. (2011). Social media in medical education: Two innovative pilot studies. *Medical Education, 45,* 1158–1159.

Gupta, S., Wan, F.T., Hall, S.E., & Straus, S.E. (2012). An asthma action plan created by physician, educator and patient online

collaboration with usability and visual design optimization. *Respiration, 85,* 406–415.

Hojat, M., Nasca, T.J., Erdmann, J.B., Frisby, A.J., Veloski, J.J., & Gonnella, J.S. (2003). An operational measure of physician lifelong learning: Its development, components, and preliminary psychometric data. *Medical Teacher, 25,* 433–437.

Hojat, M., Veloski, J.J., & Gonnella, J.S. (2009). Measurement and correlates of physicians' lifelong learning. *Academic Medicine, 84,* 1066–1074.

Jaffar, A.A. (2014). Exploring the use of a Facebook page in anatomy education. *Anatomical Sciences Education, 7,* 199–208.

Kind, T., Patel, P.D., & Lie, D. (2013). Opting in to online professionalism. *Pediatrics, 132*(5), 792–795.

Kind, T., Patel, P.D., Lie, D., & Chretien, K.C. (2014). Twelve tips for using social media as a medical educator. *Medical Teacher, 36,* 284–290.

Knowles, M.A., Holton, E.F, Swanson, R.A. (2005). *The Adult Learner: The Definitive Classic in Adult Education and Human Resource Development* (6th ed.). Burlington, MA: Elsevier.

Kolb, D.A. (1984). *Experiential Learning,* Englewood Cliffs, NJ: Prentice Hall.

Lanning, L.C., & Dadiq, B.A. (2010). A strategy for incorporating palliative care and end-of-life instruction into physician assistant education. *Journal of Physician Assistant Education, 21,* 41–46.

McAndrew, M., & Johnston, A. (2012). The role of social media in dental education. *Journal of Dental Education, 76,* 1474–1481.

McGowan, B.S., Wasko, M., Vartabedian, B.S., Miller, R.S., Freiherr, D.D., & Abdolrasulnia, M. (2012). Understanding the factors that influence the adoption and meaningful use of social media by physicians to share medical information. *Journal of Medical Internet Research, 14*(5):e117.

Merriam, S.B., & Caffarella, R.S. (1999). *Learning in Adulthood: A Comprehensive Guide.* San Francisco, CA: Jossey-Bass.

Mezirow, J. (1990), How Critical Reflection triggers Transformative Learning. In J. Mezirow & Associates (eds), *Fostering Critical Reflection in Adulthood: A Guide to Transformative and Emancipatory Learning.* San Francisco, CA: Jossey-Bass, pp. 1–20.

Pew Research Center. (2014). Pew Research Center Internet Project January Omnibus Survey. Retrieved from http://www.pewinternet.org/fact-sheets/social-networking-fact-sheet/

Pinilla, S., Weckbach, L.T., Alig, S.K., Bauer, H., Noerenberg, D., Singer, K., & Tiedt, S. (2013). Blogging medical students: A qualitative analysis. *GMS Zeitschrift für Medizinische Ausbildung, 30,* Doc9.

Priem J, Groth P, Taraborelli D (2012). The altmetrics collection. *PLoS ONE, 7*(11), e48753.

Sandars, J., Homer, M., Pell, G., & Croker, T. (2008). Web 2.0 and social software: The medical student way of e-learning. *Medical Teacher, 30,* 308–312.

Schön, D.A. (1990). *Educating the Reflective Practitioner: Toward a New Design for Teaching and Learning in the Professions.* San Francisco, CA: Jossey Bass.

Sunderland, N., Camm, C.F., Glover, K., Watts, A., & Warwick, G. (2014). A quality assessment of respiratory auscultation material on YouTube. *Clinical Medicine, 14*(4), 391–395.

Taylor, D.C. & Hamdy, H. (2013). Adult learning theories: Implications for learning and teaching in medical education: AMEE Guide No. 83. *Medical Teacher, 35*(11), e1561–1572.

Topps, D., Helmer, J., & Ellaway, R. (2013). YouTube as a platform for publishing clinical skills training videos. *Academic Medicine, 88,* 192–197.

Tower, M., Latimer, S., & Hewitt, J. (2014). Social networking as a learning tool: Nursing students' perceptions of efficacy. *Nurse Education Today, 34,* 1012–1017.

Wang, A.T., Sandhu, N.P., Wittich, C.M., Mandrekar, J.N., & Beckman, T.J. (2012). Using social media to enhance continuing medical education: A survey of internal medicine CME course participants. *Mayo Clinic Proceedings, 87,* 1162–1170.

Wang, T., Wang, F., & Shi, L. (2013). The use of microblog-based case studies in a pharmacotherapy introduction class in China. *BMC Medical Education, 13,* 120.

Wetzel, A.P., Mazmanian, P.E., Hojat, M., Kreutzer, K.O., Carrico, R.J., Carr, C., ... Rafiq, A. (2010). Measuring medical students' orientation toward lifelong learning: A psychometric evaluation. *Academic Medicine, 85*(Suppl.10), S41–44.

Yardley, S., Teunissen, P.W., & Dornan, T. (2012). Experiential learning: Transforming theory into practice. *Medical Teacher, 24,* 161–164.

Live tweeting in medicine: 'Tweeting the meeting'

ALEXANDER M. DJURICICH & JANINE E. ZEE-CHENG

Indiana University School of Medicine, Indianapolis, Indiana, USA

Abstract

Medical conferences create an opportunity for lifelong learning for healthcare practitioners. The use of Twitter at such conferences continues to expand. This article focuses on how Twitter can be used by physicians and other healthcare providers at regional, national and international conferences, and also at local conferences, such as grand rounds. It also addresses the potential utility of Twitter chats and journal clubs in the promotion of lifelong learning. The impact of Twitter use in healthcare in general, and specifically at conferences, and how it can be measured, is discussed.

Introduction

Little is constant in medicine except its evolution. Science progresses, practice changes, techniques are refined; healthcare practitioners must commit to lifelong learning to adapt to these changes. Another paper in this supplement covers the intersection of social media with personal and professional development and lifelong learning (Kind, pp. 00–00).

The venues for lifelong learning are not limited to classrooms or textbooks. Local educational sessions such as grand rounds provide an opportunity for learning that can be streamlined into a daily schedule. Healthcare practitioners at all levels attend these sessions, and they are invaluable to medical education. On a national and international level, large speciality conferences are a place for like-minded practitioners to gather and share knowledge. Conferences are crucial for many specialities as a way to encourage academic activities and stay abreast of current literature in order to optimize patient outcomes (Davis et al., 1999). Although there are some opportunities at grand rounds and larger conferences for interaction, these conversations tend to be 'face-to-face' before or after formal learning sessions. With the introduction of Twitter, some of the barriers to engagement and interaction at conferences have started to break down (Chaudhry et al., 2012).

The aim of this paper is to provide a synthetic review of the literature that currently exists about tweeting at conferences. We will first briefly describe Twitter and how it works. We will then review articles that describe results of Twitter use at local, regional, national, and international conferences. We will also address the use of Twitter to facilitate journal clubs and topical chats. We will discuss outcomes as defined by different authors and will also address possible future utility and significance of 'tweeting the meeting'.

Background

The advent of Twitter in 2006 introduced an unfamiliar social environment. This new form of largely public conversation in which 'short bursts of inconsequential information' (Sano, 2009) are relayed in 140-character 'tweets' seemed an unlikely home for lifelong learning. Yet as Twitter became more popular, its users – physicians, medical journals, and medical organizations (Kamel Boulos & Anderson, 2012) – began to realize its utility in acquiring and distributing medical information. McGowan et al. wrote that physicians use social media platforms such as Twitter to 'contribute knowledge, to seek it, and to scan and explore (McGowan et al., 2012). In addition, social media is used by practitioners to communicate with professional colleagues (Antheunis et al., 2013). Indeed, descriptions of how to use Twitter in clinical practice have made their way into mainstream medical literature (Melvin & Chan, 2014). Twitter becomes, then, a conference of sorts – a meeting of the minds online, rather than in an exotic locale. At its core Twitter is a way for healthcare practitioners to connect, communicate, and share knowledge, potentially across vast geographic distances. Sending out tweets during conferences ('tweeting the meeting') helps to unify this virtual public classroom, as do Twitter chats and journal clubs.

Twitter terminology

Box 1.

@[username]	Identifies individual users. Usernames are always preceded by the '@' sign. Usernames may or may not be the 'real life' name of a user. For example, Alex Djuricich's username is @MedPedsDoctor; Janine Zee-Cheng's username is @JanineZeeCheng.
Mention	To include a username in a tweet, i.e. 'According to @JanineZeeCheng, antibiotics should not be used to treat viral infections.'
Hashtag	A searchable word, phrase, abbreviation, or acronym preceded by a hash or number sign, e.g. '#AAP14'. Users add the hashtag onto individual tweets; doing so provides the ability to unify all related tweets into one coherent timeline
Retweet	The posting of a user's tweet by another user who finds it helpful or useful
Live tweet	To tweet in real-time, e.g., during a lecture or a conference

How Twitter works

Individual users create profiles on the Twitter website, and are then able to compose and publish 140-character tweets in real time. Tweets may contain nearly any content: for example, text, hashtags, mentions, photos, or links to other websites. An example of a tweet containing both hashtags and mentions might be:

@JanineZeeCheng: Just completed PC3 conference on #palliativecare #endoflife care by @gbosslet @lfettig. What a GREAT experience!

Users may 'follow' one another. For example, if @MedPedsDoctor follows @JanineZeeCheng, the above tweet will appear on @MedPedsDoctor's Twitter home page. This home page contains a timeline of real-time tweets from everyone that @MedPeds-Doctor follows.

Tweeting grand rounds

Grand rounds are an educational tradition within academic medicine (Sandal et al., 2012). Weekly or monthly presentations are attended by medical students, residents, fellows, and faculty staff in medical schools worldwide. Despite its academic distinction, the educational value of grand rounds has been questioned: some have suggested increasing the use of technology to foster enhanced engagement with audience members (Lewis, 2012).

One such enhancement might be adding a second screen at grand rounds presentations; one screen displays the content, the other shows a live Twitter stream viewed by the participants. A viewable Twitter feed provides three benefits: a way for non-users to learn about Twitter, a forum for interaction about the topic being discussed, and the ability to contribute knowledge to interested Twitter users who are not in attendance. Some have even described Twitter as a 'backchannel' for alternative discussions about the content (Ross et al., 2011).

At our children's hospital we studied the impact of this during a series of grand rounds within the Department of Pediatrics at the Indiana University School of Medicine (Djuricich, 2014). We used the hashtag '#IUPedsGrRounds'. Seventeen consecutive grand rounds presentations were tweeted by audience participants. A total of 613 tweets occurred during those 17 presentations, for a mean of about 35 tweets per hour-long grand rounds session. We classified themes of the grand rounds into clinical topics, Education topics, Research topics, Quality Improvement/Patient Safety topics, and Advocacy topics. The topics under the advocacy theme had the highest number of tweets per session, while those under the research theme had the lowest. Since that time, a variety of faculty and resident members continue to tweet the grand rounds content. Future study of similar educational interventions such as this can determine how best to disseminate information to learners.

Tweeting international, national, and regional conferences

At medical society conferences the use of Twitter has increased, and medical associations are now beginning to recognize the power of Twitter as a form of information dissemination (Neill et al., 2014). A number of specialities have published outcomes from using Twitter at their national conferences. Chaudhry et al. described an 83% increase in number of tweets and a 2.4 fold increase in physician Twitter users from the American Society of Clinical Oncology (ASCO) national meeting between 2010 and 2011 (Chaudhry et al., 2012). Subsequently, Matta et al. analysed the number of tweets from the American Urological Association (AUA) and Canadian Urological Association (CUA) national meetings between 2012 and 2013 and found that in a single year there was a 5-fold increase in both the volume of tweets and the number of urologists who contributed to the online conversation about the annual meetings (Matta et al., 2014). Wilkinson et al. recently analysed Symplur metrics from eight urology conferences and demonstrated a dramatic increase in Twitter use; the number of Twitter participants at the European Annual Congress increased 10-fold over a 3-year period (from 2012–2014), and the number of tweets went from 347 to almost 6,000 (Wilkinson et al., 2014).

Significance lies not only in the increasing number of healthcare practitioners using Twitter at meetings; the content of such tweets also matters. There have been a number of studies that address the educational content of tweets from national conferences. Chaudhry et al. found that at the ASCO national meeting, 26% of tweets contained links to articles or references related to the meeting; in 2011, the number was 22% (Chaudhry et al., 2012). Matta et al. found that 39% of AUA and CUA tweets were considered informative by a classification scheme devised by the authors (Matta et al., 2014). Jalali et al. analysed tweets from the 2013 Canadian Conference on Medical Education (CCME) and found that Twitter was used to discuss the medical education themes related to the conference, which supported the idea that Twitter may be a useful tool for facilitating discussions related to conference topics (Jalali et al., 2013).

Because one of the benefits of Twitter is the ability to communicate with users across geographic distances, the reach of informative content also matters. Neill et al. described Twitter use at the 2012 International Conference on Emergency Medicine and found that although over 400 people authored tweets about the conference, only 34% of these people were actually physically in attendance. Further, 74.4% of these tweets were directly related to the material presented at the conference (Neill et al., 2014). Similar findings have been found in other specialities, such as surgery, in which just 19 of the 37 tweet authors were in attendance at the 2013 Academic Surgical Conference (Cochran et al., 2014). Mishori et al. found that one of the reasons for using Twitter at the 2013 Society of Teachers of Family Medicine conference was sharing information with others, particularly those not in attendance (Mishori et al., 2014). Table 1 highlights publications on the use of Twitter at national medical conferences. The effective use of Twitter at conferences has even been described in other non-medical scientific journals (Ekins & Perstein, 2014).

However, while it may be claimed that social media has significantly altered the conference experience (Wilkinson et al., 2014), the true impact of this form of communication, and subsequent learning, is difficult to quantify. Measurable tools include hashtags, which, as described previously, allow pooling of related content from a particular meeting. Communications and public relations offices within societies will often create buzz around a hashtag before the meeting: 'Don't forget to follow conference tweets at the hashtag '#AAP14' (for the 2014 National Conference and Exhibition of the American

Table 1. Description of articles describing the use of Twitter at national conferences.

Author	Year	Speciality field	Hashtag	Metric	Highlights
Mishori et al. (2014)	2014	Family medicine	#STFM13	Tweets: 1,818 Tweet authors: 181	Twitter can be used as a 'conversation starter' among like-minded individuals
Neill et al. (2014)	2014	Emergency medicine	#ICEM12	Tweets: 4,692 Tweet authors: 401	Conference content reached a significant number of Twitter users not physically attending
Cochran et al. (2014)	2014	Surgery	#2013ASC	Tweets: 434 Tweet authors: 58	Twitter team of four responsible for 76% of all tweets. Organizers should develop a social media strategy for conferences
Jalali & Wood (2013)	2013	Medical education	#CCME13	Tweets: 3,090 Tweet authors: 288	Conference organizers should implement new innovations that would facilitate use of social networking tools
Matta et al. (2014)	2014	Urology	#AUA13 #CUA13	Tweets: 4,591 Tweet authors: 540	Compared 2012–2013 data. Use by urologists dramatically shifted between 2012 and 2013
Wilkinson et al. (2014)	2014	Urology	#EUA13 #USANZ13 #AUA13 #BAUS13 #CUA13 #PCWC13 #ERUS #SIU2013	Tweets: 12,363 Tweet authors: 1,592	Twitter use by urologists has increased significantly at many national and international meetings
Desai et al. (2012)	2012	Nephrology	#kidneywk11	Tweets: 993 Tweet authors: 172	An ideal tweet would include three features: 1) informative content; 2) internal citations; 3) positive sentiment score
Chaudhry et al. (2012)	2012	Oncology	#ASCO10 #ASCO11	Tweets (by physicians): 12,644 Tweet authors: 48	Compared 2011 data to 2010. Twitter use grew significantly between 2010 and 2011. Professional societies should monitor these phenomena to enhance annual meeting attendee user experience

Academy of Pediatrics). The company Symplur has created the online 'Healthcare Hashtag Project' (Symplur, 2014a). With this tool, hashtags can be registered, and usage data extracted and analysed. Analytics include the number of tweets within a specified time period, the 'top tweeters' of a hashtag, and number of mentions of a particular user. Symplur metrics were used in a number of the studies referenced here; this resource provides a way to measure the reach of a particular hashtag. Despite the non-peer-reviewed nature of tweets, the number of tweets produced after an article is published may predict future citations (Eysenbach, 2011). Another similar tool is AltMetrics, a tool used to capture the impact of articles by tracking them when they are mentioned online, such as in blogs or social media platforms (Brigham, 2014). AltMetrics was developed as a complement to traditional article citation analyses, but its use has expanded beyond articles to analyse other scholarly endeavours (Priem et al., 2012).

Etiquette

The literature on the etiquette of tweeting during conferences is sparse (Cordell, 2014). Online editorials on the topic describe specific ways to optimize interaction without significant interruption for other learners. A focus on maintaining professional boundaries is of utmost importance when tweeting at conferences.

Are conference speakers even aware that tweeting is occurring? Some may be reluctant to allow tweeting during their presentations, but if the goal of conference presentations is to disseminate information, the use of Twitter as a viable form of communication of content should be considered. Conference organizers have reminded speakers that their content may be tweeted by participants. Some conference managers may ask that participants not tweet material during the presentation, and conference attendees should honour such requests. Cochran et al. suggested that other courtesies include encouraging appropriate attribution of findings to the speakers, withholding tweets about any research presented that is under embargo pending publication, and limiting tweeted photographs of slides used in the presentation (Cochran et al., 2014).

While there is no established standard for providing attribution for tweets when 'tweeting the meeting', it stands to reason that appropriate credit and citation should be included in the tweet. For example, the hashtag for the 2015 American Psychiatry Association annual conference might be '#APA2015', and a fictional speaker named Francis Peabody might state: 'The secret in caring for the patient is in the care of the patient' (Peabody, 1984). A tweet from a participant in the conference could be as follows:

@MedPedsDoctor: F Peabody. The secret in caring for the patient is in the care of the patient. #APA15

With the increasing popularity of live tweeting, some social media experts have even offered advice about how to effectively tweet a meeting. Suggestions include recruiting a team of volunteers and having them attend rehearsals beforehand in order to effectively broadcast the most important aspects of the session (Reissman, 2014).

Twitter chats and journal clubs

Live tweeting does not have to occur during a formal presentation; it can also occur during a twitter chat. Chats, like other Twitter interactions, are conversations between users. They take place at a specified time, and a facilitator guides the flow of conversation so users stay on topic. Because Twitter is a public space, anyone interested may participate – from high school students to healthcare providers. The 'community of practice' nature of Twitter (Lewis & Rush, 2013; Ranmuthugala et al., 2011) is reflected in the healthcare communications and social media (#hcsm) chat. Participants include clinicians, patients, family members, researchers, and journalists. This particular chat has a venerable history; created in 2009 by communications expert Dana Lewis, who also self-discloses as having type 1 diabetes mellitus, it now has an enthusiastic following and generates lively discussion weekly. A chat on the topic of medical education, #meded, began in 2011 and often brings educators, medical students, residents, fellows and patients together for a robust discussion on a variety of medical education topics (Colbert & Chokshi, 2014), not only at the undergraduate medical education level, but also at the graduate and continuing education levels. These chats are transcribed into a chronological timeline so the conversation can be easily read and revisited (Madanick, 2014).

Like Twitter chats, journal clubs may occur in real time at a predetermined time; alternatively, they may be asynchronous over a day or two. Articles are selected ahead of time and announced by the facilitator, and questions are addressed and answered under a dedicated hashtag. Online journal clubs have been described in other fields including paediatrics (Webber et al., 2013), internal medicine (Mehta & Flickinger, 2014), and emergency medicine (Rolston & Lee, 2014). Twitter provides a new virtual classroom for these discussions to take place; it bridges geographic barriers and brings together participants with diverse experiences and perspec-

Table 2. Examples of Twitter chats and journal clubs in medicine.

Username	Hashtag	Description
@HealthSocMed	#hcsm	Healthcare communications and social media chat. Sundays 8pm Central Standard Time
@MedEdChat	#meded	Medical education chat. Thursdays 9pm Eastern Standard Time
[no username assigned; chat is by hashtag only]	#pulmCC	Pulmonary and critical care medicine chat. Monthly
@psychiatryjc	#psychjc	Psychiatry journal club. Asynchronous, third Wednesday of each month
@nephjc	#nephjc	Nephrology journal club. Asynchronous. Also at NephJC.com
@iurojc	#urojc	Urology journal club. Asynchronous, first Sunday/Monday of each month

tives (Mehta & Flickinger, 2014). Table 2 provides examples of different Twitter chats and journal clubs in varying medical specialities.

Challenges

Despite the potential positives which social media can provide, challenges to its meaningful use within medicine still exist. Lapses in professionalism around social media are common in the lay literature, and have been described within medicine as well (Chretien et al., 2011; Strausburg, 2011). The American College of Physicians, in conjunction with the US Federation of State Medical Boards, has outlined social media use guidelines, but it is up to each individual user to abide by them (Farnan et al., 2013). Panahi et al. describe other challenges to social media use among healthcare practitioners. These include maintaining confidentiality, lack of active participation, lack of trust of other social media users, finding time, workplace acceptance and support, and 'information anarchy' – the lack of control of information management and data flow (Panahi et al., 2014). In addition, some may join the social media conversation, but the honeymoon phase is not permanent, and interest can fade for a variety of reasons (Glyde, 2014).

The best and worst aspect of Twitter is that it is a public space with a diverse population. Healthcare practitioners are present, but so are many other users, whose attention may be caught momentarily by a particular hashtag, leading to a perhaps irrelevant commentary on an established topic. Even conferences tweeted by a designated Twitter team were noted to have a significant proportion of non-academic (social or promotional) tweets (Cochran et al., 2014). Also, online Twitter chats and journal clubs sometimes attract participants whose only intention seems to be to disrupt the conversation.

Although these challenges are significant, a cadre of healthcare practitioners are tweeting (Lee et al., 2014), and many have meaningful messages for the recipients of those tweets. Participants all over the world now have the power to incorporate a limitless online classroom into their individualized learning networks. By leveraging tools such as Twitter to disseminate information from medical conferences, participants can utilize another avenue for the acquisition, contribution, and dissemination of knowledge that can be put into practice for the optimal care of patients.

Perhaps because of more prevalent social media engagement among healthcare practitioners, there appears to be increased interest in scholarly investigation of the impact of social media within medicine. Fox et al. published the first randomized trial assessing the impact of social media use (Fox et al., 2014). It was found that a social media strategy did not increase the number of page views of articles in a cardiovascular journal. Interestingly, while the study found no impact of a social media strategy, discussion of the article generated around 300 tweets during a one hour Twitter medical education chat on 20 November 2014 (Symplur, 2014b).

While there is little academically rigorous literature to support the educational benefit of 'tweeting the meeting', various social media strategies – the Amyotrophic Lateral Sclerosis (ALS) Ice Bucket Challenge (Wicks, 2014), for example, or using the influence of Twitter as a tool for influenza surveillance (Aslam et al., 2014; Pawelek et al., 2014) – can demonstrate the potential impact of social networking on medical research and public health. Future implications and next steps might be to consider evaluating educational and potentially patient-level outcomes from the use of Twitter at conferences.

Conclusion

Lifelong learning is an integral part of any healthcare professional career that can be facilitated by attendance at medical association conferences, whether local, regional, national, or international. Conference attendance, in turn, can be enhanced by the use of social media platforms such as Twitter. Although the impact of 'tweeting the meeting' requires future study, current and ongoing research suggests that social media's role in medicine, like medicine itself, continues to evolve in today's technology-driven, ever-connected world.

Acknowledgements

The authors would like to thank Emily Webber for useful discussions and encouragement regarding tweeting grand rounds.

Declaration of interest: The authors report no conflicts of interest. The authors alone are responsible for the content and writing of the paper.

References

Antheunis, M.L., Tates, K., & Nieboer, T.E. (2013). Patients' and health professionals' use of social media in health care: Motives, barriers and expectations. *Patient Education and Counseling, 92*, 426–431.

Aslam, A.A., Tsou, M.H., Spitzberg, B.H., An, L., Gawron, J.M., Gupta, D.K., … Lindsay, S. (2014). The reliability of tweets as a supplementary method of seasonal influenza surveillance. *Journal of Medical Internet Research, 16*, e250.

Brigham, T.J. (2014). An introduction to altmetrics. *Medical Reference Services Quarterly, 33*, 438–447.

Chaudhry, A., Glode, M.L., Gillman, M., & Miller, R.S. (2012). Trends in Twitter use by physicians at the American Society of Clinical Oncology annual meeting, 2010 and 2011. *Journal of Oncology Practice, 8*, 173–178.

Chretien, K.C., Azar, J., & Kind, T. (2012). Physicians on Twitter. Research letter. *Journal of the American Medical Association, 35*, 566–568.

Cochran, A., Kao, L.S., Gusani, N.J., Suliburk, J.W., & Nwomeh, B. (2014). Use of Twitter to document the 2013 Academic Surgical Congress. *Journal of Surgical Research, 190*, 36–40.

Colbert, J.A., & Chokshi, D.A. (2014). Technology in medical education – Osler meets Watson. *Journal of General Internal Medicine, 29*, 1584–1585.

Cordell, R. (2014). Mea culpa: On conference tweeting, politeness and community building. *Chronicle of Higher Education.* Retrieved from http://chronicle.com/blogs/profhacker/mea-culpa-on-conference-tweeting-politeness-and-community-building/45861

Davis, D., O'Brien, M.A., Freemantle, N., Wolf, F.M., Mazmanian, P., & Taylor-Vaisey, A. (1999). Impact of formal continuing medical education: Do conferences, workshops, rounds, and other traditional continuing education activities change physician behavior or health care outcomes? *JAMA, 282*, 867–874.

Desai, T., Shariff, A., Shariff, A., Kats, M., Fang, X., Christiano, C., & Ferris, M. (2012). Tweeting the meeting: An in-depth analysis of Twitter activity at Kidney Week 2011. *PLoS One, 7*(7), e40253.

Djuricich, A.M. (2014). Social media, evidence-based tweeting and JCEHP. *Journal of Continuing Education in the Health Professions, 34*, 202–204.

Ekins, S., & Perlstein, E.O. (2014). Ten simple rules of live tweeting at scientific conferences. *PLOS Computational Biology, 10*, e1003789.

Eysenbach, G. (2011). Can tweets predict citations? Metrics of social impact based on Twitter and correlation with traditional metrics of scientific impact. *Journal of Medical Internet Research, 13*, e123.

Farnan, J.M., Snyder Sulmasy, L., Worster, B.K., Chaudhry, H.J., Rhyne, J.A., & Arora, V.M. (2013). Online medical professionalism: patient and public relationships: policy statement from the American College of Physicians and the Federation of State Medical Boards Special Committee on Ethics and Professionalism. *Annals of Internal Medicine, 158*, 620–627.

Fox, C.S., Bonaca, M.P., Ryan, J.J., Massaro, J.M., Barry, K., & Loscalzo, J. (2014). A randomized trial of social media from Circulation. *Circulation, 131*, 28–33.

Glyde, T. (2014). Social media: Toxified by rage. *Lancet Psychiatry, 1*, 337–338.

Jalali, A., & Wood, T.J. (2013). Tweeting during conferences: Educational or just another distraction? *Medical Education, 47*, 1129–1130.

Kamel Boulos, M.N., & Anderson, P.F. (2012). Preliminary survey of leading general medicine journals' use of Facebook and Twitter. *Journal of the Canadian Health Libraries Association, 33*, 38–47.

Lee, J.L., DeCamp, M., Dredze, M., Chisolm, M.S., & Berger, Z.D. (2014). What are health-related users tweeting? A qualitative content analysis of health-related users and their messages on Twitter. *Journal of Medical Internet Research, 16*, e237.

Lewis, B., & Rush, D. (2013). Experience of developing Twitter-based communities of practice in higher education. *Research in Learning Technology, 21*, 18598.

Lewis, D.W. (2012). Are pediatric grand rounds dead? *Journal of Pediatrics, 160*, 711–712.

Madanick, R.M. (2014, 20 November). #MedEd chat transcript. Retrieved from https://drive.google.com/file/d/0ByRfWmxlYdoYbFBGWXM5WUtJdU0/view

Matta, R., Doiron, C., & Leveridge, M.J. (2014). The dramatic increase in social media in urology. *Journal of Urology, 192*, 494–498.

McGowan, B.S., Wasko, M., Vartabedian, B.S., Miller, R.S., Freiherr, D.D., & Abdolrasulnia, M. (2012). Understanding the factors that influence the adoption and meaningful use of social media by physicians to share medical information. *Journal of Medical Internet Research, 14*, e117.

Mehta, N. & Flickinger, T. (2014). The times they are a-changin': Academia, social media and the JGIM Twitter Journal Club. *Journal of General Internal Medicine, 29*, 1317–1318.

Melvin, L., & Chan, T. (2014). Using Twitter in clinical education and practice. *Journal of Graduate Medical Education, 6*, 581–582.

Mishori, R., Levy, B., & Donvan, B. (2014). Twitter use at a family medicine conference: analyzing #STFM13. *Family Medicine, 46*, 608–614.

Neill, A., Cronin, J.J., Brannigan, D., O'Sullivan, R., & Cadogan, M. (2014). The impact of social media on a major international emergency medicine conference. *Emergency Medicine Journal, 31*, 401–404.

Panahi, S., Watson, J., & Partridge, H. (2014). Social media and physicians: Exploring the benefits and challenges. *Health Informatics Journal, 2014*. doi: 10.1177/1460458214540907.

Pawelek, K.A., Oeldorf-Hirsch, A., & Rong, L. (2014). Modeling the impact of Twitter on influenza epidemics. *Mathematical Biosciences and Engineering, 11*, 1337–1356.

Peabody, F.W. (1984). Landmark article March 19, 1927: the care of the patient. By Francis W. Peabody. *JAMA, 252*, 813–818.

Priem, J., Groth, P., & Taraborelli, D. (2012). The Altmetrics collection. *PLoS ONE, 7*, e48753.

Ranmuthugala, G., Plumb, J.J., Cunningham, F.C., Georgiou, A., Westbrook, J.I., & Braithwaite, J. (2011). How and why are communities of practice established in the healthcare sector? A systematic review of the literature. *BMC Health Services Research, 11*, 273.

Reissman, H. (2014). How-to: 7 steps to creating a dynamic livetweeting strategy for your event. Retrieved from http://tedxinnovations.ted.com/2014/11/26/how-to-7-steps-to-creating-a-dynamic-livetweeting-strategy-for-your-event

Rolston, D.M., & Lee, J. (2014). Annals of Emergency Medicine Journal Club. Is it still cool to cool? Interpreting the latest hypothermia for cardiac arrest trial: Answers to the March 2014 Journal Club questions. *Annals of Emergency Medicine, 64*, 199–206.

Ross, C., Terra, S.M., Warwick, C., & Welsh, A. (2011). Enabled backchannel: Conference Twitter use by digital humanists. *Journal of Documentation, 67*, 214–237.

Sandal, S., Iannuzzi, M.C., & Knohl, S.J. (2012). Can we make grand rounds 'grand' again? *Journal of Graduate Medical Education, 5*, 560–563.

Sano, D. (2009, February 18). Twitter creator Jack Dorsey illuminates the site's founding document. *Los Angeles Times.* Retrieved from http://latimesblogs.latimes.com/technology/2009/02/twitter-creator.html

Strausburg, M. (2011). How Facebook almost ended my career with a single click. *Academic Emergency Medicine, 18*, 1220.

Symplur. (2014a).Symplur Healthcare Hashtag Project. Retrieved from http://www.symplur.com/healthcare-hashtags/

Symplur. (2014b). Symplur #meded social media analytics for 20 November 2014. Retrieved from http://www.symplur.com/healthcare-hashtags/MedEd/analytics/?hashtag = MedEd&fdate = 11%2F20%2F2014&shour = 18&smin = 00&tdate = 11%2F20%2F2014&thour = 19&tmin = 01

Webber, E., Saysana, M., & McKenna, M. (2013). Journal club blog for faculty paediatricians. *Medical Education, 47*, 1128.

Wicks, P. (2014). The ALS ice bucket challenge: Can a splash of water invigorate a field? *Amyotrophic Lateral Sclerosis and Frontotemporal Degenerations, 15*(7–8), 479–480.

Wilkinson, S.E., Basto, M.Y., Perovic, G., Lawrentschuk, N., & Murphy, D.G. (2014). The social media revolution is changing the conference experience: Analytics and trends from eight international meetings. *BJU International*, 2014. doi: 10.1111/bju.12910.

Social media and medical education: Exploring the potential of Twitter as a learning tool

ALIREZA JALALI[1], JONATHAN SHERBINO[2], JASON FRANK[2] &
STEPHANIE SUTHERLAND[1]

[1]*Faculty of Medicine, University of Ottawa, Ottawa, Ontario,* [2]*The Royal College of Physicians and Surgeons of Canada (RCPSC), Ottawa, Ontario, Canada*

Abstract

This study set out to explore the ways in which social media can facilitate learning in medical education. In particular we were interested in determining whether the use of Twitter during an academic conference can promote learning for participants. The Twitter transcript from the annual International Conference on Residency Education (ICRE) 2013 was qualitatively analysed for evidence of the three overarching cognitive themes: (1) preconceptions, (2) frameworks, and (3) metacognition/reflection in regard to the National Research Council's (NRC) How People Learn framework. Content analysis of the Twitter transcript revealed evidence of the three cognitive themes as related to how people learn. Twitter appears to be most effective at stimulating individuals' preconceptions, thereby engaging them with the new material acquired during a medical education conference. The study of social media data, such as the Twitter data used in this study, is in its infancy. Having established that Twitter does hold significant potential as a learning tool during an academic conference, we are now in a better position to more closely examine the spread, depth, and sustainability of such learning during medical education meetings.

Introduction

Social media is changing the world as we know it. Contemporary medical education is reflective of this global paradigm shift. Definitions of social media are diverse, including a focus on e-learning and distance education learning tools, and narrower interpretations include the discussions of websites and applications where users contribute, retrieve, and explore content primarily generated by fellow users (McGowan et al., 2012). Recently social media use as a learning tool in medicine has been growing at an exponential rate. It can build on e-learning in ways that are more learner-generated, collaborative, and engaging (Batt-Rawden et al., 2014). The basic idea of Twitter is to follow users' tweets and write one's own. By following interesting chains of messages and commenting on them, users can collect enthusiastic followers. One of Twitter's most recognizable features is hashtags, expressed with the symbol #. Hashtags are Twitter's own way of pointing out keywords, and through them it is possible to follow a certain theme or event. Clicking on a hashtag lets the user see all the tweets related to that subject (Auvinen, 2013).

As an online social networking service, Twitter can be accessible from any Internet-capable device. While other social networking sites are online confessionals or portfolios of personal current events, Twitter is designed and used as a vehicle to converse and share ideas (Forgie et al., 2013). For this reason, we postulate that Twitter may hold much potential as a learning tool for medical education. This type of knowledge sharing or microblogging has been found to have broad value as a news and communication medium, but little is known about the process of knowledge acquisition (Kwak et al., 2010). Previous studies have tended to focus on extremes such as retweeting and unfollowing (Andre et al., 2012).

In a previous study an analysis was conducted on information dissemination using Twitter during the 2013 Canadian Conference on Medical Education (CCME), which is the largest meeting of this type in Canada. The guiding research question was, 'Are tweeters chatting about medical education topics related to the conference or just creating a background of white noise?' (Jalali & Wood, 2013). The results showed that Twitter was used to discuss the medical education themes related to the conference more often than for any other purposes. This supports the idea that Twitter may be a useful tool for facilitating discussions related to conference topics. From this initial study we wanted to probe deeper to obtain a better understanding of how learning can take place using Twitter as a social medium during a medical education conference. Thus, the purpose of the current study is to analyse the Twitter transcript's content value and its related uses during an academic meeting. Our focus was to utilize an evidence-based approach to analyse the Twitter dataset from the 2013 annual International Conference on Residency Education (ICRE). Broadly speaking, the goals of ICRE are to utilize the conference as a global forum for those involved in residency education to share ideas and innovations as well as to advance medical education. Studying the potential of Twitter as a mechanism for social capital during the ICRE 2013 annual meeting can provide a snapshot of how learning may be acquired and shared among participants.

Background

Twitter as a social medium

The use of social media has spread rapidly in the past few years, as demonstrated in increasing numbers of users, types of media, mobile applications, and connectivity. The power of social media to affect society is based exclusively on its social aspects: this means interaction and participation. Undeniably, we live in an increasingly social world, and it is social capital that underlies all social relations. Social capital has been described as an actual and potential resource embedded in relationships among actors, and increasingly it is seen as an important predictor of group and organizational performance (Adler & Kwon, 2002). Social capital is used to describe the nature of relations among organizational members, as well as the relations between the organization and its external stakeholders, competitors, and/or partners. In particular, social capital is broken down into two parts: internal and external social capital. Internal social capital permits us to look inside an organization and examine relationships among individual members or groups (Coleman, 1988). Coleman pointed to one particularly important property that he called the degree of closure within social structures and networks. Closure in this sense refers to the extent of interconnectedness among group members. By contrast, external social capital focuses on the external relations between the organization and its important stakeholders (Coleman, 1990). Twitter as a social medium provides a unique opportunity to examine how social capital, both internal and external, is dispersed within a community of users within a particular domain.

The American Society of Nephrology (ASN) has turned to social media, namely Twitter, to uses its annual conference to inform and educate the public about kidney disease. Since the dissemination of information is necessary if Twitter is to be considered a tool to increase public awareness of kidney disease, a study was undertaken to analyse tweets during the official 2011 Kidney Week conference. Through linguistic content analysis, the authors found that Twitter can be used to disseminate educational information about kidney disease if the tweets had three key features: informative content, internal citations, and a positive sentiment score (calculated through content analysis of each tweet) (Desai et al., 2012). Similarly, Letierce et al. (2010) explored how Twitter was used during a particular conference with the following hashtag: '#iswc2009'. The main outcome was that on one hand, one can make sense of tweets to identify what happened during the conference, and on the other hand, in spite of a general willingness to share outside their community, the current tagging habits direct the messages mainly to their peers.

The power of social media to affect society is based exclusively on its social aspects: this means interaction and participation. Social constructivists purport that learning is fundamentally a social phenomenon, reflecting our own deeply social nature as human beings (Wenger, 1998). The primary focus of this theory of learning is social participation, and the power of social media to affect society is based on these same principles of social interaction, namely interaction and participation. However, our educational institutions are largely based on the assumption that learning is an individual process. The purpose here is not to debate the theoretical underpinnings of knowledge generation but rather to start at the level of the individual before moving to the group and/or community level. Thus, to better understand how individuals, in this case conference participants internalize knowledge, we turn to the psychological literature as structural guideposts for the necessary construction of meaning.

Psychological foundations of individual learning

By learning, we mean more than the simple acquisition of knowledge. Rather, we mean learning as the construction of meaning by the learner (Prawat, 1996). Knowledge is created and re-created on the basis of previous learning through the search for personal meaning-making (Bruning et al., 1999). The National Research Council's synthesized report on how people learn discusses three overarching cognitive themes that rest on a solid research base that can be taken to explicate the process of meaning-making as referenced above (Brandsford et al., 1999; Donovan & Bransford, 2000). A simplified version is listed below:

1. Individuals hold preconceived notions about given content domains. If these initial understandings

are not engaged, individuals may fail to grasp the new concepts and information to which they are exposed.

2. To develop competence in a given domain, individuals must have a foundation of declarative and procedural knowledge and understand these ideas in the context of a conceptual framework that facilitates this application.

3. 'Metacognitive', or reflective, opportunities can help individuals take control of their own learning by defining goals and monitoring the progress toward achievement.

Readers who are interested in the theoretical and empirical underpinnings of the aforementioned themes are encouraged to consult the full report (Donovan, 2000). For now, we take the three 'key findings' as an operational definition of the process of individual learning and use them to determine whether learning is accomplished by using Twitter at a medical education conference.

Methods

Twitter is a relatively new social medium, and its use in social science research methods, and more broadly in higher education, is in its infancy. Researchers are experimenting with different approaches to analyse the 'Twitter metrics' gleaned from datasets. A promising approach is to utilize typologies and categorize tweets from qualitative linguistic content analysis methods (Andre et al., 2012; Desai et al., 2012; Naaman et al., 2010). For this study we sought to establish Twitter as a learning tool within the psychological literature before turning our attention to the creation, use, and modification of typologies as a further frame for this programme of research. Qualitative coding methods were applied to the #ICRE2013 Twitter dataset (Miles & Huberman, 1994). In the current study we utilized all participant tweets during the official conference time frame. The unit of analysis is the individual. Each tweet from the #ICRE2013 transcript was qualitatively coded by two of the authors (S.S. & A.J.) for evidence of the NRC's three cognitive themes of preconceptions, frameworks, and metacognition/reflection. In an ongoing practice of ensuring trustworthiness in our data analysis we instituted an inter-rater reliability check. To establish inter-rater reliability in our coding, each coder codes the same transcript and comes together for a consensus meeting. That is, the two coders need to agree on the codes assigned to the transcript text. In tandem, a codebook is created to record the codes whereby consensus has been achieved, with a definition and reference to the text. The process continues, transcript by transcript until the raters achieve 80% agreement within the codes

assigned to the text (Teddlie & Tashakkori, 2009). To assist with the retrieval and organization of this data, we used Symplur (see www.symplur.com).

By 2014 more than 400 healthcare conferences have registered their hashtag with Symplur. Symplur has the largest database of healthcare conversations on Twitter today with more than 180 million tweets, all categorized by over tens of thousands of healthcare topics (Symplur, 2014). Symplur is a tool that can, among other things, collect healthcare conference Twitter data and produce both a transcript of tweets as well as perform analytics. Among the 373 ICRE 2013 conference participants, there were 4,958 tweets during the conference (26–28 September 2013). This resulted in an average of 34 tweets per hour with 4,815,052 impressions. The Symplur platform is also able to list the top influencers by the Twitter name and associated total number of tweets during the conference.

Results

The large majority of healthcare conferences have spikes in tweet activity during conference days. Analysis of peak Twitter activity during #ICRE 2013 is indicative of this trend, namely peaks in activity occurring around noon on each day (see Fig. 1). Analysis of the tweets revealed the content areas of presentations occurring on given conference days. For example, 27 September had the highest number of tweets, surpassing 900 tweets. As illustrated in Fig. 1, conference sessions of particular interest on that day (marked with an X) included career-spanning ePortfolio, CanMEDS, and entrustable professional activities (EPAs) to name a few. This type of analytical visual is important in understanding what topics were of most interest to participants. Next we will delve into the cognitive dimensions of learning that resulted from the Twitter activity.

Application of the 'How People Learn' Framework

Preconceptions. Prototypical evidence of what can be described as a cultivation of awareness within participants has been discovered. The quote excerpts suggest an increase in consciousness of a disparity between the current state of affairs and a suggested alternative. Reviewing the Twitter transcript for the #ICRE 2013 meeting, one finds a developing awareness of the divergence of topics applicable to resident training. Tweets coded under the preconceptions theme included:

Can Twitter activity be used to evaluate audience engagement? Does more tweets from the crowd = a better session? (27 September @ 9:54 am)

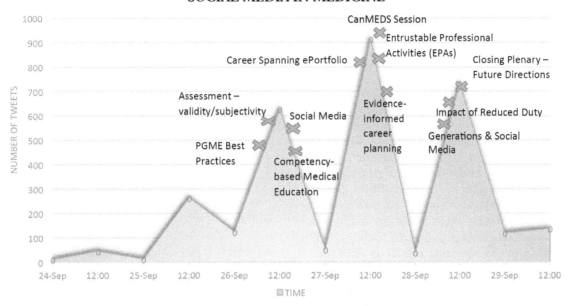

Fig. 1. #ICRE content of tweet activity during conference.

Competency once achieved is not competency maintained. (27 September @ 13:02 pm)

Assessment is a diagnostic test. Assessment should be used in an integrative way for action. Maintain a healthy mistrust of numbers. (28 September @ 8:40 am)

Entrustable professional activity – descriptors of practice rather than the individual. (28 September 13:15 pm)

Being on social media is not a popularity competition, it's identity management. (28 September @ 10:30 am)

This first cognitive theme yielded the highest number of coded tweets of the three cognitive themes. It can be postulated that much of the information-gathering during the conference sessions is new and/or is challenging individuals to incorporate this new information with their pre-existing preconceptions of particular knowledge domains. In many instances it appears that this is the first encounter for individuals to begin to engage with these new ideas. The tweet, 'Can Twitter activity be used to evaluate audience engagement? Does more tweets from the crowd = a better session?' is indicative of someone trying on a new perspective with respect to the evaluation of sessions using Twitter.

Frameworks

Frameworks speak to the issue of structuring knowledge. A hallmark of cognitive psychology is an emphasis on knowledge organization. Knowledge structures direct perception and attention, permit

comprehension, guide recall, and facilitate application. In their review of research in this domain, Bruning et al. (1999) highlighted the instructional implications of this theme and advocated for the use of 'tools for understanding' such as analogies, metaphors, and various other organizing frameworks. The Twitter discourse reflects conference participants' experiences with some of the different organizers they encountered while at the conference. Conference participants also acknowledged the utility of organizing frameworks that came by way of guiding questions, thus providing structure to their newly acquired knowledge.

Can Entrustable Professional Activities (EPAs) serve as measures of competency milestones? (27 September @ 10:10 am)

What to do when a candidate fails a CanMEDS competency? Interesting discussion. (27 September @ 12:00 pm)

Teaching strategies from Master teachers – Teach according to the level of the learner and the time available. (27 September @ 13:02 pm)

Can't get away with competency-based icing on a time-based cake. (28 September @ 14:05 pm)

The individual who tweeted 'What to do when a candidate fails a CanMEDS competency? Interesting discussion' has demonstrated attention to the issue (namely of failing a competency), recall is operationalized by referencing the CanMEDS framework, and the pre-existing guide of the CanMEDS framework helps to structure the thought processes of the activities surrounding failure. And, the tweet 'Can't get away with competency-based icing on a time-based cake' is a good example of participants coming to terms with new paradigms and using an analogy to organize information.

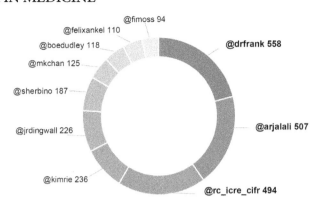

Fig. 2. #ICRE 2013 influencers by number of mentions.

Metacognition/reflections

This third cognitive theme yielded the fewest coded tweets. This could be, in part, due to the real-time nature of Twitter, and one would postulate that reflection would occur in the near future. Schon's concept of reflection-in-action refers to an individual's conscious thought about his or her actions and the thinking that accompanies them (Schon, 1987). In reviewing the Twitter data one finds evidence of participants' reflections on their own learning. That is, participants engage in a conscious interpretation of past events in relation to new learning.

> Making EPAs – Think of your practice and think about what must be done every week. (27 September @ 12:17 pm)

> The number one thing that can make us good leaders is being mindful of what we're doing and reflecting for improvement. (28 September @ 14:20 pm)

> Good presentations by residents on duty hours and 'impact' of reduction in hours. Hot topic here. More discussion needed. (28 September @ 12:32 pm)

Influencers: promoters of knowledge

Another interesting dimension of Twitter analytics is the display of the influencers. That is, to what degree do key individuals assist in developing, leading, and sustaining conversation? Twitter analytics revealed the highest number of conference influencers by the number of mentions in the dataset (see Fig. 2). It is evident that the users @drfrank 558, @arjalali 507 and @rc_icre_cifr 494 were the highest influencers. This data is important in terms of discovering who the key leaders are. In this way, Twitter can be used as an influence generator in creating waves of influence through original posts and selective re-tweeting at a medical conference. These leaders contribute heavily to the community, and they contribute to the critical mass of the conversation, but more importantly the community can rely on these individuals to keep the conversation going and increase the robustness of the ongoing activity.

Upon examining the top 10 influencers, we found that the strength of these presenters and their ideas was clearly revealed in the analysis of who these top influencers were. In analyzing the top three influencers

by number of Twitter mentions, it is not surprising that two of the authors are recognized in this category as both are strong advocates of the use of social media in medical education. Also, we observed many new users each morning and afternoon, suggesting a host of new activity regarding interests and points of view.

Discussion

Analysis of tweets during a conference can produce a 'trail' of what happened during a conference. Fig. 1 was illustrative that the 'peaks' in Twitter usage occurred at approximately noon on each of the conference days. Also, Twitter can be a good way to capture the small nuggets of information you glean while at a conference. Indeed, not all tweets during a conference hold learning value: many 'bursts' of tweets appeared to have value for social communication and awareness (the equivalent of saying 'great job' after a presentation) rather than for any substantive content in terms of educational learning.

Ultimately, change must occur first at the level of the individual before we can begin to think more broadly about organizations and social communities. This study has provided a starting point for the potential learning that social media such as Twitter can have. Preconceptions appear to be the most salient acquisition of new knowledge, though we did find examples of the use of frameworks, and to a lesser extent evidence of metacognition/reflection. Perhaps following the tweets after the conference is over, for example thirty days after the official end of the meeting, could shed more light if participants continue to engage and reflect on conference ideas and points of interest.

Twitter can be an ideal tool to use as a broker for impact. For example, this type of social media has the potential to influence both internal and external social capital. That is, one or two posts from a medical conference may point hundreds of people to information they never would have sought on their own. One way to learn how a community operates is to find out about key members who have the potential to influence tone, topic, or policy for the whole community. A community organizer may be one such actor, but for a community to operate robustly, actions associated with keeping the community or the conversation going need to be distributed to more than one person (Grudz & Haythornthwaite, 2013).

Limitations

This study set out to examine the potential of Twitter as a mechanism for social capital during the ICRE 2013 annual meeting. We postulated that Twitter may be valuable for participants to acquire and share knowledge during an academic conference. It must be acknowledged that the degree to which participants learning improved via the use of Twitter cannot be determined by this qualitative study. Future work could include a randomized study whereby conference participants could be more closely examined and outcome could be tracked. Further, we do not precisely know the impact that our top influencers had on both internal and external conference participants but this is an area that we would like to probe further. Overall, this study has provided much enthusiasm among the research team to explore innovative ways of analysing Twitter datasets to determine how learning takes place but also how far-reaching it can be. Next we present some of the many interesting directions this research can take.

Next steps

With further research and applications of media literacy, Twitter is likely to become a useful tool for more personalized teaching and learning in medical education. Social media networks such as Twitter and Facebook provide exciting opportunities that, according to a recent issue of the American Sociological Association journal (*ASA Footnotes*), can 'open up a new era' of social science research (Golder & Macy, 2012). Research using social media to extract information to understand behaviours and learning approaches is in its infancy. The potential for this research has yet to be realized. Below we lay out some possible avenues for ongoing research in this area.

First, examining Twitter as a conversation starter during an academic conference could yield insights into how far a particular idea/comment can travel. For example, if someone posts an interesting point, people at the conference and those not at the conference may find that point interesting too and may ask a question and engage in further discussion. The use of Twitter analytics can assist with determining the depth, spread, and sustainability of such ideas.

Second, performing ongoing, in-depth analysis with regard to tweet content would provide further development and refinement of typologies and categorization of tweets. For example, Naaman et al. (2010) developed a 'tweet categorization scheme' which includes categories like 'Me Now' (current mood or activity), 'Presence Maintenance' (e.g. Hello Twitter), 'Self-Promotion' (e.g. sharing a blog post the author just published), and 'Information Sharing'. While such categories may not necessarily lend themselves to medical education conference content, they are useful starting points in developing an academic-oriented typology.

Third, by utilizing social network analysis we can obtain a better understanding of engagement and collaboration by examining community leaders, their positions (e.g. centrality in the community), and the impact of their influence. Three social network measures can be used to locate influential individuals in this community: (1) the total number of messages contributed during a given time frame (e.g. a conference), (2) the number of times a person is mentioned or is replied to, that is, their @username is used in a post by someone else (in-degree centrality), and (3) the number of times a person mentions or replies to others, that is, an individual uses another person's @ username in a post (out-degree centrality) (Grudz & Haythornthwaite, 2013).

Further, there appears to be a need to expand the use of qualitative methods to analyse Twitter datasets. In particular, the brevity of the messages, coding at the super-ordinate level seems most reasonable and practical. However, uses of finer-grained linguistic analysis may prove effective (Lacity & Janson, 1994). Finally, we need to better understand the network structure that facilitates and sustains learning. We need a better understanding of value and knowledge generation/transmission. For example, further research could delve into the area of digitally mediated social network actors' attributes (Adamic & Adar, 2003; Eagle et al., 2007; Leskovec & Horvitz, 2007).

Declaration of interest: The authors report no conflicts of interest. The authors alone are responsible for the content and writing of the paper.

References

Adamic, L., & Adar, E. (2003). Friends and neighbors on the web. *Social Networks*, 25(3), 211–230.

Adler, P., & Kwon, S. (2002). Social capital: Prospects for a new concept. *Academy of Management Review*, 27, 17–40.

Andre, P., Bernstein, M., & Luther, K. (2012). Who gives a tweet? Evaluating microblog content value. Paper presented at the Computer Supported Cooperative Work Conference, Seattle, WA, 11–15 February, Retrieved from https://www.cs.cmu.edu/~pandre/pubs/whogivesatweet-cscw2012.pdf

Auvinen, A. (2013). Suomen Toivo – Think Tank: Social media – The new power of political influence version 1.0. Brussels: Centre for European Studies.

Batt-Rawden, S., Flickinger, T., Weiner, J., Cheston, C., & Chisolm, M. (2014). The role of social media in clinical excellence. *Clinical Teacher, 11*(4), 264–269.

Brandsford, J., Pellegrino, J., & Donovan, S. (1999). *How People Learn*. Washington, DC: National Academy Press.

Bruning, R., Schraw, G., & Ronning, R. (1999). *Cognitive Psychology and Instruction.* Upper Saddle River, NJ: Merrill.

Coleman, J. (1988). Social capital in the creation of human capital. *American Journal of Sociology, 94*, 95–120.

Coleman, J. (1990). *Foundations of Social Theory*. Cambridge, MA: Belknap Press.

Desai, T., Shariff, A., Shariff, A., Kats, M., Fang, X., Christiano, C., & Ferris, M. (2012). Tweeting the meeting: An in-depth analysis of Twitter activity at Kidney Week 2011. *Plos One, 7*(7), 40253.

Donovan, M.S., & Bransford, J.D. (2000). Scientific inquiry and how people learn. *In M.S. Donovan & J.D. Bransford (Eds), How Students Learn: History in the Classroom. Washington, DC: National Academies Press. Retrieved from* http://www.nap.edu/catalog/11100.htm

Eagle, N., Pentland, A., & Lazer, D. (2007). Inferring friendship network structure by using mobile phone data. *Proceedings of the National Academy of Sciences, 106*(36), 15274–15278.

Forgie, S., Duff, J., & Ross, S. (2013). Twelve tips for using Twitter as a learning tool in medical education. *Medical Teacher, 35*, 8–14.

Golder, S., & Macy, M. (2012). Social science with social media. *ASA Footnotes, 40*(1), 7.

Gruzd, A., & Haythornthwaite, C. (2013). Enabling community through social media. *Journal of Medical Internet Research, 15*(10), e248.

Jalali, A., & Wood, T.J. (2013). Tweeting during conferences: Education or just another distraction? *Medical Education, 47*, 1119–1146.

Kwak, H., Lee, C., Park, H., & Moon, S. (2010). What is Twitter, a social network or a news media? Proceedings of the WWW10 Conference, Raleigh, NC, 26–30 April (pp. 591–600). New York: ACM. Accessed at http://dl.acm.org/citation.cfm?id=1772751.

Lacity, M., & Janson, M. (1994). Understanding qualitative data: A framework of text analysis methods. *Journal of Management Information Systems, 11*(2), 137–155.

Leskovec, J., & Horvitz, E. (2007). Worldwide buzz: Planetary-scale views on an instant-messaging network. Proceedings of the 17th international conference on world wide web, New York, NY, USA.

Letierce, J., Passant, A., Breslin, J., & Decker, S. (2010). Using Twitter during an academic conference: The #iswc2009 use-case. Paper presented at the International AAAI Conference on Weblogs and Social Media, Washington, DC, 23–26 May. Retrieved 9 October 2014 from https://www.aaai.org/ocs/index.php/ICWSM/ICWSM10/paper/view/1523/1877

McGowan, B., Wasko, M., Vartabedian, B., Miller, R., Freiherr, D., & Abdolrasulnia, M. (2012). Understanding the factors that influence the adoption and meaningful use of social media by physicians to share medical information. *Journal of Medical Internet Research, 14*(5), e117.

Miles, M., & Huberman, A. (1994). *Qualitative Data Analysis: An Expanded Sourcebook*. Thousand Oaks: SAGE.

Naaman, M., Boase, J., & Lai, C. (2010). *Is it really about me? Message content in social awareness streams. Paper presented at the CSCW10 Conference, Savannah, GA, 6–10 February.*

Prawat, R.S. (1996). Constructivism, modern and post-modern. *Educational Psychologist, 31*, 215–225.

Schon, D. (1987). *Educating the Reflective Practitioner*. San Francisco: Jossey-Bass.

Symplur. (2014). Analyzing twitter conversations from health-care conferences. Retrieved from http://www.symplur.com/blog/analyzing-twitter-conversations-from-healthcare-conferences

Teddlie, C., & Tashakkori, A. (2009). *Foundations of Mixed Methods Research: Integrating Quantitative and Qualitative Approaches in the Social and Behavioural Sciences*. Thousand Oaks, CA: Sage

Wenger, E. (1998). *Communities of Practice*. Cambridge: Cambridge University Press.

Social media, medicine and the modern journal club

JOEL M. TOPF[1] & SWAPNIL HIREMATH[2,3,4]

[1]Oakland University William Beaumont School of Medicine, Rochester, Michigan, United States of America,
[2]Renal Hypertension Unit, Division of Nephrology, Department of Medicine, University of Ottawa, Ontario, Canada,
[3]Ottawa Hospital Research Institute, Ottawa, Ontario, Canada, and [4]Hypertension Unit, Division of Cardiology,
University of Ottawa Heart Institute, Ottawa, Ontario, Canada

Abstract

Medical media is changing along with the rest of the media landscape. One of the more interesting ways that medical media is evolving is the increased role of social media in medical media's creation, curation and distribution. Twitter, a microblogging site, has become a central hub for finding, vetting, and spreading this content among doctors. We have created a Twitter journal club for nephrology that primarily provides post-publication peer review of high impact nephrology articles, but additionally helps Twitter users build a network of engaged people with interests in academic nephrology. By following participants in the nephrology journal club, users are able to stock their personal learning network. In this essay we discuss the history of medical media, the role of Twitter in the current states of media and summarize our initial experience with a Twitter journal club.

Introduction

The field of education is rapidly changing, and this change has accelerated in the last few years (Kahn et al., 2014). As these changes accumulate, they pose an existential threat to the conventional bricks-and-mortar model of learning. Some believe medical education is protected from these changes, but in the last 50 years medical education has also witnessed multiple disruptions in the textbooks, journals, study guides and other media that support it (henceforth termed medical media). The arc of change has tracked across multiple axes:

- improved search
- reductions in price
- simplification in production

Each of these axes has direct benefits to the user, and the products that introduced significant leaps in any of one of them have been able to establish footholds in physician education. It is not yet clear how far these still-evolving changes will take us, or how much they will end up revolutionizing the field of medical education. In this essay we provide our personal and idiosyncratic overview of these advances. In some of these we have been interested bystanders, but more recently we have become active instigators.

In the beginning

The modern story of medical media begins with Tinsley Harrison disrupting the market for internal medicine textbooks. Harrison's *Principles of Internal Medicine* (Pittman, 2011) was not the first textbook of medicine and at the time of publication, Cecil's was the pre-eminent textbook. Harrison brought two important innovations to the field. Cecil, like all other contemporary medicine texts, was organized by disease, offering the definition, cause, symptoms, treatment, and prognosis for each malady. This meant that to use the book, doctors first needed to have a diagnosis; Harrison's *Principles of Internal Medicine*, in contrast, introduced a symptom-based and regional organization to the book. The ability to look up abdominal pain and see the myriad of diseases that could be the cause made Harrison's more useful for both the novice and practising physicians. In addition to being a practical book, Harrison's emphasized the biological basis of disease and is credited as being the first textbook to break down the wall between basic science and clinical medicine (DuBois, 2007).

Being digital

Four decades after the first edition of Harrison's, Burton D. Rose began publishing his landmark internal medicine text book on CD-ROM, UpTo-Date, Post TW (Ed). Rose wrote the text in stages building from organ to organ, and speciality to speciality. He recruited top medical scientists from every speciality and over the course of a decade produced a comprehensive database of medicine, marrying an internal medicine textbook to comprehensive coverage of paediatrics, surgery and obstetrics. UpToDate (Waltham, MA) brought a number of innovations to medical media, but the central tent pole was 'search'. Instant access on a computer meant no more pulling an ancient tome from your shelf and trudging through the index.

The break from text also meant that the tyranny of the page limit could finally end. Previously, textbooks began with a target page number based on the presumed retail price. Based on that price the maximum number of pages was set. The editor distributed those pages across the various chapters, authors and subjects. Any new diseases or concepts the editor wanted to include necessarily meant decreasing coverage of other areas. Rose's natively digital text eliminated these external limits. New diseases and additional concepts never compromised other sections. Loss of page limits allowed increased depth of coverage that was never available in previous medical textbooks. UpToDate up-ended the textbook market by being fast, comprehensive and deep (Rose, 2013).

Biggest price drop ever

After the CD-ROM came the Internet and online resources. The defining characteristic of this revolution was the price, free*. Standouts of this revolution include MedScape, WebMD, and ePocrates (Table 1). Each was free and each offered a different type of content.(Benigeri & Pluye, 2003; McMullan, 2006) Though the content is free, these are for-profit companies, producing professional content, written by experts. The biggest difference from previous generation's medical media is that the money no longer comes from the readers, but rather from advertisers. Because there is money being exchanged, we refer to this price as being free with an asterisk, or 'free*'.

A side effect of pairing 'search' and 'free' is a radical democratization of medical information. Patients, families, medical students, nurses, and doctors are, for the first time, playing on the same information playground; everyone has access to the same information.

Here comes everybody

After free* came 'the crowd in the cloud'. Wikipedia is the prototypical example of a crowd-sourced information site and in medicine it is the only example that matters. Jimmy Wales rustled up an army of 70,000 editors and set out to write about ... well everything (Wikipedia, 2014).

Wikipedia is at, or near, the top of most Google searches of medical terms, and that hallowed spot generates a lot of traffic (Fig. 1). Our residents, medical students and peers are going to Wikipedia. Though the lure of the top link in a Google is powerful, if the information does not answer the question, clever medical students and residents would quickly route around useless Wikipedia links. That is not happening. The proof that the information in Wikipedia is 'good enough' is that residents, students and doctors keep going back to use it (Allahwala et al., 2013; Beck, 2014; Morris, 2013; Namdari, 2011). Despite resistance from established stakeholders in medical education, Wikipedia continues to gain momentum and recently some structured efforts to improve the quality of Wikipedia have emerged, with medical students earning credit for improving medical Wikipedia pages (Cohen, 2013; Wikipedia, 2013).

Another form that the crowd in the cloud arrived in was e-mail subscriptions, often called listservs. Based on technology from the last century, users send an e-mail to a single address which rebroadcasts the e-mail to all of the subscribers to the list. Replies to the initial e-mail would similarly be rebroadcast to everyone (Caropreso, 2014). By using e-mail, this technology exploited a distribution network that is both easy to understand and universally deployed around the world. E-mail lists are able to bring geographically diverse populations with narrow interests together. The Nephrol list, founded and run by Kim Solez, is still actively sharing information among nephrologists (Solez, 2014). One of the major advantages was that one could pick the brains of the foremost experts internationally (John Daugirdas, Jim Tattersall and the late Dimitrios Oreopoulos to name a few) who are part of the network. However, the weakness in the technology comes from the problem of scalability – as more and more people participate in the discussion e-mail boxes become clogged, causing people to unsubscribe from the list.

Push button publishing for the people

The latest innovation in the medical media is the medical blog with information shared through social

Table 1. Examples of free medical media that emerged during the late 1990s' dot.com boom.

MedScape	News, commentary, clinical information
WebMD	Patient oriented, symptom decoder
ePocrates	Point of care drug information
eMedicine	Medical textbook

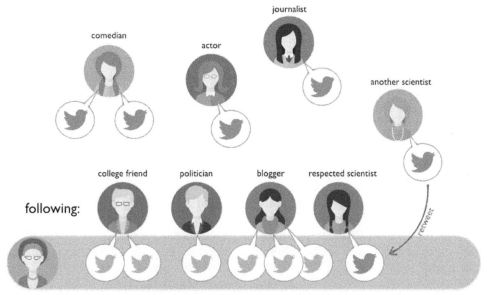

Your timeline only shows tweets of the people you follow.

When people you follow retweet other users you will then
see tweets from users you do not follow on your timeline

Fig. 1. The timeline displayed in the native Twitter app. Twitter displays tweets from accounts you follow. Tweets from other accounts will only show up in your timeline if one of the people you follow retweets a specific tweet from someone else.

platforms (Cadogan, 2014). The medical blog erupted in popularity when web publishing became so simple and easy that it could be done for free with online tools. Blogger and Wordpress.com removed the technical barriers to online publishing. If you could use Microsoft Word you had all the essential skills needed to publish your thoughts to the world. Blogs allowed countless doctors to become medical journalists and commentators. Some doctors gathered audiences of other doctors while others gained lay audiences of patients seeking health information. Others specialized in public policy. Two prominent examples are:

- Kevin Pho, a New Hampshire family practitioner began blogging in 2004. He has turned this blog into one of the centres of medical blogging, with over 1,000 bloggers, mostly doctors, contributing to his blog. His success in the online world has catapulted him to widespread prominence as a physician commentator to both physician and mainstream audiences (AAMC, 2014).
- Aaron Carroll has used blogging to publicize his well-researched health policy and to promote his books of medical minutia and myth busting. He began blogging in 2009 and this blogging ultimately led to him writing for CNN, *JAMA*, and the *New York Times*. He says blogging is the most valuable thing he does (personal communication).

Blogging allows the great medical explainers to have audiences larger than three residents and two bored medical students from the rounding team

(Garrity et al., 2014). However, discovery remains a problem. Most individual blog posts get swallowed in the ocean of the World Wide Web and are rarely read. Dr Topf's nephrology blog has nearly 700 posts but only a dozen or so have any appreciable traffic from Google search. Typical nephrology searches (hyponatraemia, dialysis, chronic kidney disease (CKD)) have large professional websites clustered on the first few pages of Google results. Indeed, the dominant source of traffic to medical blogs turn out to be direct links from Twitter. The social network of short text snippets is the modern form of peer review and word of mouth. This is not a unique experience, and has been noted by others (Terras, 2012). Indeed, most journals have joined Twitter, and tweet links to their articles. Adding to the frenzy was the discovery that the volume of tweeting in the first three days after publication was predictive of future citations. Tracking tweets provides the earliest clue to which papers are destined to have high impact (Eysenbach, 2011).

The problem with Twitter

Twitter is the first social network designed from the outset for mobile. The 140-character limit was designed to allow an entire tweet to fit into a single SMS message (Bilton 2013a). It is malleable to fulfil many needs. It can be a news wire service, it is the contemporary dial-a-joke, it can be used to follow friends. In medicine, however, it is being used to recommend and endorse articles, opinions and posts from a wide swath of primary sources (Lee et al., 2014). It can be an answering machine, able to deliver diverse solutions, usually complete with references from the literature, within minutes of asking.

However, if free open access medical resources represented democratization of information, Twitter goes one step further to sometimes appear as anarchy. Unlike Google search, Twitter has no hierarchy of established or trusted sources of information. The limited palette of options, just 140 characters of text, a link or two and maybe a picture, means that large, sophisticated organizations have no compelling way to differentiate themselves from talented individuals – both play on the same level playing field. Anne-Marie Slaughter, an advisor to Secretary Clinton explained, 'A seventeen-year-old with a smartphone can now do what it used to take an entire CNN crew to do' (Bilton, 2013b).

Harnessing the power of Twitter and taming the anarchy of information requires grooming a careful cohort of people to follow. Since publishing to Twitter is so effortless, the site is thick with meaningless navel gazing and celebrity drivel. Getting value requires cultivating a useful and engaging network. Since the value of Twitter is related to the sophistication of one's network, it is difficult for new users to see much utility in the product. Bridging that gap between the value experienced users receive and the lack of apparent value to the new user has been a recurring question in medical social media. What was needed was a way for people to quickly build an effective community, or personal learning network (PLN), in order for Twitter to provide value (Siemens, 2005; Edublogs Teacher Challenges, 2014).

#NephJC, a nephrology journal club on Twitter

One way to jumpstart the creation of a PLN is holding an event that brings engaged, high-value people together. It is the online equivalent of the residency picnic during orientation week. A picnic that brings everyone out together, neophytes and old-hands, so people everywhere can mix and build their networks. In order to gather an audience of nephrologists interested in medical education, the event needed to be just right, i.e. a Monday night football chat would not attract the right people.

The event that the authors created is a twice monthly Twitter-based journal club examining the most interesting studies, editorials, reviews and clinical practice guidelines driving the practice of nephrology. The event is called NephJC. NephJC works like a Twitter chat, a live, moderated discussion centred on a single topic (Cooper, 2013). Chats are tied together with a unique hashtag. NephJC uses #NephJC. Hashtags are metadata that describe the subject of the tweet, they also work as search terms and filters. A conference hashtag like #Med20 tell users that the Tweet has something to do with the Med 2.0 Conference and #Ferguson indicates the tweet is about the riots over St Louis County Policing. Clicking on a hashtag in Twitter will conduct a search of all tweets that contain that hashtag. This search filters out other tweets and fundamentally changes the usage model of Twitter.

In the standard use of Twitter, users only see the tweets of people they follow (Fig. 2). This model bends if one of the people the user is following republishes a tweet from another user (retweet, in the vernacular of the service), in that case one would see that tweet despite not following the original author. If a user, however, clicks on a hashtag, or uses specialized software optimized to follow hashtags (e.g. Tweet-Chat.com, tchat.io, TweetDeck), the user will see all the tweets tagged with the selected hashtag of interest, regardless of whether one follows the author or not. At the same time, while using the hashtag-selective software, the user will no longer see the tweets of the people she follows unless they use the hashtag. The hashtag thus focuses attention on a topic of interest, and one can follow all commentaries from the Twittersphere on that particular topic (Fig. 3). This is less useful when following a hashtag of national interest, but for a relatively niche area, like a nephrology journal club, it is transformative. The hashtag allows users to break out of their own timeline and see how people they do not follow are participating in the discussion. This is a catalyst to developing one's PLN because it lets people see all the people tweeting on this esoteric but important (to the nephrologist) topic.

The journal club chat actually begins about a week before the discussion, when an announcement of the next article is posted to NephJC.com. NephJC.com is the web home for the Twitterchats. The website keeps archives of previous chats and also serves to store pertinent background material for the chats. Soon after the announcement, we update the website with some context and summary of the article. As the organizers of NephJC, we cajole and enlist other nephrology bloggers to post additional commentary, background or context. This serves to promote the chat and broaden the audience. Renal Fellow Network, Precious Bodily Fluids, AJKDblog, Nephrology On-Demand, Nephron-Power and Whizzbang have all participated in extending and promoting the chats. Over the following week the organizers tweet about the study, linking to related literature, editorials and related news stories. Part of the build-up includes an e-mail to a growing list of subscribers. The e-mail serves to notify people who use Twitter less frequently and may otherwise miss these promotions.

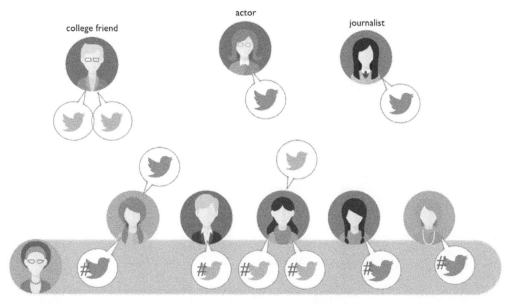

When you follow a hashtag, instead of seeing the tweets of people you follow you will see all the tweets with the hashtag and only the tweets with the hashtag.

Fig. 2. When a user either clicks on a #hashtag, or uses specialized software to follow a #hashtag (e.g. tchat.io, TweetChat, TweetDeck), the user will see all the tweets tagged with that #hashtag, whether the user follows them or not. In this interface, one also does not see tweets from the accounts one follows, unless they are tagged with that particular #hashtag, allowing the attention to be focused on that particular topic.

The discussion begins at the appointed hour. Anyone interested is welcome – nephrologists, other specialists, trainees from all levels, and patients. The talk is hosted by the NephJC Twitter account, which is operated by one of the creators. The host prepares a few talking points and attempts to guide the conversation. The chats are free-wheeling with opinions and ideas spinning into multiple conversation threads. The chat is typically a mix of thoughtful questions, clever answers, nerdy jokes and a number of references and links to the medical literature. Some participants come prepared with data, citations and images and provide a lot of free open access meducation, or FOAMed (#FOAMed is a hashtag that tags medical media as free and open access), others bring clinical experience, while others bring a sharp wit to enliven the proceedings. The turnout has ranged from 13 to 60 people. We suspect that some number of additional users follow the

Impressions	9,075,683
Tweets	6,655
Participants	603

Fig. 3. A summary of Symplur analytics for #NephJC for the period from March to October 2014. The 'impressions' figure is calculated by multiplying the number of tweets with the number of followers that account has. A more nuanced discussion of these analytics is available at http://www.nephjc.com/nephjc-the-first-dozen/.

conversation, but do not join the discussion by tweeting. These participants are invisible and uncountable, e.g. lurkers. Despite not tweeting, they presumably still gain value from passively watching and reading along. The cast of people participating in each chat varies from day to day so that after 16 chats, 603 people participated (Fig. 4).

After the hour-long chat concludes, the organizers compile a complete transcript of the chat, which is made available at NephJC.com. Since this is not always easy to follow with the sheer number of tweets (in the range of 200–300 tweets per session), an edited version of the chat is also made available. This curated transcript is created using a tool called Storify and on occasion there are multiple Storifies made for a single chat, as different individual curators select different tweets to represent the chat.

The summaries, links to the original article, the transcript and curated transcripts are all compiled on a single web page. A short summary of the conclusions of the journal club and a link to the page is posted on the article's PubMed page using NLM's social tool, PubMed Commons (http://www.ncbi.nlm.nih.gov/pubmedcommons/). This makes the NephJC discussion available to people who find the article through PubMed (see this link for an example: http://www.ncbi.nlm.nih.gov/pubmed/25244096 #cm25244096_7171).

There are several other advantages to using Twitter for an activity like a journal club. Twitter has avoided

	Wikipedia	NIH	MedScape	WebMD	PubMed	CDC	UpToDate	Med journal	.org	.com
central pontine myelinolysis	2	1	3					5,6	7,8	4
Unstable Angina	4	1	5,6	9				10	2,7,8	3
Neprilysin	1				3,4			2,5,8,10	6,7	9
APACHE score	1		2		5		7	6,10	3	4,8,9
Lithium toxicity	2	1	3				8			4,5,6,7,9,10
Neuroleptic malignant syndrome	1	2	3	4			5	9,10	6	7,8
extrapyramidal symptoms	1		2	6	3					4,5,7,8,9,10
BRCA1	2	1,3,4						5,6,7,8,9,10		
Lynch Syndrome	4	1				6			2,7,8,9	5,10
Autism spectrum disorder	3	1		2		5			6,7,8,9	10
C. Diff	2	3			1	4			5,6,7,10	8,9

Fig. 4. This screenshot shows the rank of various sites in the list of Google results when searching for the term in the first column. Note: Google gives different results for different users depending on history, location, and other information not made public. This test was done while logged out of Google to get as unbiased a result as possible.

the privacy pitfalls entangling Facebook by boiling down the privacy equation to complete simplicity: everything on Twitter is public, nothing is private (actually there are some corners of Twitter, specifically direct messaging, that are private, and people can lock their accounts in order to attempt some semblance of privacy, but the primary use case for the service entails an open and public data trail). The lack of privacy means that while one is tweeting journal club thoughts, the remainder of one's followers see these tweets and the hashtag and often spontaneously join the conversation. These spontaneous participants often bring fresh perspectives from specialities outside of nephrology or outside of medicine entirely. Also, by not being limited to a single institution, a broader range of skills often show up to join the chat. Christos Argyropoulos is a nephrologist with advanced training in statistics and brings valuable perspective often not available in many face-to-face journal clubs. On occasion, one of the study authors joins the discussion, providing a unique insight into study design and rationale.

In our social implementation of the traditional journal club we have taken the opportunity to broaden the scope of what is typically examined in journal club. At times we have used NephJC to draw attention to documents that, while not research articles, needed careful evaluation. We dissected the hyponatraemia guidelines produced by a consortium of the European Society of Intensive Care Medicine, the European Society of Endocrinology and the European Renal Association – European Dialysis and Transplant Association (Spasovski et al., 2014). Clinical practice guidelines are determining more and more of how we practice medicine and deserve the same scrutiny previously reserved for research articles. We also have discussed editorials, another document typically not considered worthy of analysis in a traditional journal club. For example, Richard Johnson's discussion on the possible aetiology of the ongoing chronic kidney disease epidemic in Central America is a critical topic for nephrology and one that should not be ignored because it is not seen in North America (Johnson et al., 2014).

Twitter journal clubs are dynamic and compelling ways to build a PLN on Twitter. It should be no surprise that this format is becoming common among other medical specialities, notably #urojc for urology, #BlueJC for OB/Gyn, #MedEd (sponsored by the Journal of General Internal Medicine, @Journal-GIM) for internal medicine, and #ALiEM for emergency medicine (Thangasamy et al., 2014; Radecki et al., 2014; Mehta et al., 2014; Leung et al., 2013). Different Twitter journal clubs, have different tweaks to the model. One weakness of NephJC is that by setting a specific time for the discussion, 9 p.m. Eastern Time results in the discussion running at 2 a.m. in England and 1pm in Sydney, Australia.

UroJC has a different model that focuses on asynchronous discussion over 48 h. This allows people all over the world to participate in the discussion (Thangasamy et al., 2014).

Conclusion

The media that supports medical education continues to evolve, but over time it is moving to be simpler to produce, resulting in more people generating content. It is simultaneously becoming cheaper to consume, resulting in more people having access to sophisticated medical education resources. Overall medical literature is becoming less hierarchical and more collaborative. Twitter journal clubs generally, and NephJC specifically, embrace these trends. It is interesting that in addition to ushering in modern medical media with *Harrison's Principles of Internal Medicine*, Tinsley Harrison was also famous for hosting spirited journal clubs (Pittman, 2011). Perhaps we are merely turning full circle.

Declaration of interest: The authors are co-creators of the website, NephJC.com, the subject of this paper. They have not and do not anticipate ever profiting financially from this association. The authors alone are responsible for the content and writing of the paper.

References

AAMC. (2014).Kevin Pho, M.D. Inspiring stories: Aspiring docs. Association of American Medical Colleges. Retrieved from https://www.aamc.org/students/aspiring/inspiring-stories/267856/kevin_pho.html

Allahwala, U., Nadkarni, A., & Sebaratnam, D. (2013). Wikipedia use amongst medical students – New insights into the digital revolution. *Medical Teacher, 35*(4), 337–337.

Beck, J. (2014). Doctors' number 1 source for healthcare information: Wikipedia. Retrieved from: http://www.theatlantic.com/health/archive/2014/03/doctors-1-source-for-healthcare-information-wikipedia/284206/ (accessed 24 October 2014).

Benigeri, M., & Pluye, P. (2003) Shortcomings of health information on the Internet. *Health Promotion International, 18*(4), 381–386.

Bilton, N. (2013a). The first CEO. In Hatching Twitter: A true story of money, power, friendship, and betrayal (p. 169). New York: Penguin.

Bilton, N. (2013b). Iranian Revolution. In Hatching Twitter: A true story of money, power, friendship, and betrayal (p. 324). New York: Penguin.

Cadogan, M., Thomas, B., Chan, T., & Lin, M. (2014). Free Open Access Meducation (FOAM): The rise of emergency medicine and critical care blogs and podcasts (2002–2013). *Emergency Medicine Journal, 31*, E76–77.

Caropreso, P. (2014). ACS rural listserv: An 'underdog' success story. *Bulletin of the American College of Surgeons, 99*(7), 48–51.

Cohen, N. (2013, September 29). Editing Wikipedia Pages for Med School Credit. *New York Times*.

Cooper, S. (2013, September 30). The ultimate guide to hosting a tweet chat. *Forbes*. Retrieved from http://www.forbes.com/sites/stevecooper/2013/09/30/the-ultimate-guide-to-hosting-a-tweet-chat/

DuBois, L. (2007, October 1). Eugene Braunwald: Maestro of American Cardiology. *Lens*. Retrieved from http://www.mc.vanderbilt.edu/lens/article/?id=181.

Edublogs Teacher Challenges. (2014, 23 September). Step 1: What is a PLN? Retrieved from http://teacherchallenge.edublogs.org/pln-challenge-1-what-the-heck-is-a-pln/

Eysenbach, G. (2011). Can tweets predict citations? Metrics of social impact based on Twitter and correlation with traditional metrics of scientific impact. *Journal of Medical Internet Research, 13*(4), E1231.

Garrity, M.K., Jones, K., Vanderzwan, K.J., De la Rocha, A.B., & Epstein, I. (2014). Integrative review of blogging: Implications for nursing education. *Journal of Nursing Education, 53*(7), 395–401.

Harrison, Tinsley Randolph. (1950) Principles of Internal Medicine. Blakiston, Philadelphia, PA.

Johnson, R.J., Rodriguez-Iturbe, B., Roncal-Jimenez, C., Lanaspa, M.A., Ishimoto, T., Nakagawa, T., … Sanchez-Lozada, L.G. (2014). Hyperosmolarity drives hypertension and CKD – Water and salt revisited. *Nature Reviews: Nephrology, 10*(7), 415–420.

Kahn, M.J., Maurer, R., Wartman, S.A., & Sachs, B.P. (2014). A case for change: Disruption in academic medicine. *Academic Medicine, 89*(9), 1216–1219.

Lee, J.L., DeCamp, M., Dredze, M., Chisolm, M.S., & Berger, Z.D. (2014). What are health-related users tweeting? A qualitative content analysis of health-related users and their messages on Twitter. *Journal of Medical Internet Research, 16*(10), e237.

Leung, E., Tirlapur, S., Siassakos, D., & Khan, K. (2013). #BlueJC: BJOG and Katherine Twining Network collaborate to facilitate post-publication peer review and enhance research literacy via a Twitter journal club. *BJOG: An International Journal of Obstetrics and Gynaecology, 120*, 657–660.

McMullan, M. (2006). Patients using the Internet to obtain health information: How this affects the patient–health professional relationship. *Patient Education Counseling, 63*(1–2), 24–28.

Mehta, N., & Flickinger, T. (2014). The times they are a-changin': Academia, social media and the JGIM Twitter Journal Club. *Journal of General Internal Medicine, 29*(10), 1317–1318.

Morris, N. (2013, November 18). Wikipedia's role in medical education brings awesome promise – And a few risks. *Boston Globe*.

Namdari, M. (2011). *Is Wikipedia taking over textbooks in medical student education?* Abstract NR02–16. *New Research*. Honolulu: American Psychological Association.

Pittman, J. (2011, August 25). Tinsley Randolph Harrison – The founding editor of Harrison's Principles of Internal Medicine. *Doctors Hangout*. Retrieved from http://www.doctorshangout.com/profiles/blogs/tinsley-randolph-harrison-the-founding-editor-harrisons-principle

Radecki, R.P., Rezaie, S.R., Lin, M. (2014). Annals of Emergency Medicine Journal Club. Global Emergency Medicine Journal Club: Social media responses to the November 2013 Annals of Emergency Medicine Journal Club. *Annals of Emergency Medicine, 63*(4):490–494.

Rose, B. (2013, January 15). The UpToDate Story. Retrieved from http://www.uptodate.com/home/uptodate-story

Cecil, Russell L. A. (1927). Textbook of Medicine, by American authors. W.B. Saunders, Philadelphia.

Siemens, G. (2005). Connectivism: A learning theory for the digital age. *International Journal of Instructional Technology and Distance Learning, 2*(1):42–49.

Solez, K. (2014, October 24). Personal communication: Medical Providers Lists.

Spasovski, G., Vanholder, R., Allolio, B., Annane, D., Ball, S., Bichet, D. … Nagler, E. (2014). Clinical practice guideline on diagnosis and treatment of hyponatraemia. *European Journal of Endocrinology, 170*(3), G1–47.

Terras, M. (2012). The impact of social media on the dissemination of research: Results of an experiment. *Journal of Digital Humanities, 1*(3), e1. Retrieved from http://journalof digitalhumanities.org/1-3/the-impact-of-social-media-on-the-dissemination-of-research-by-melissa-terras/

Thangasamy, I.A., Leveridge, M., Davies, B.J., Finelli, A., Stork, B., & Woo, H.H. (2014). International Urology Journal Club via Twitter: 12-month experience. *European Journal of Urology, 66*,112–117.

Wikipedia. (2013). Wikipedia: WikiProject Medicine/UCSF Elective 2013. Retrieved from https://en.wikipedia.org/wiki/Wikipedia:WikiProject_Medicine/UCSF_Elective_2013

Wikipedia. (2014). Wikipedia: Wikipedians. Retrieved from http://en.wikipedia.org/wiki/Wikipedia:Wikipedians

A personal reflection on social media in medicine: I stand, no wiser than before

JOHN WEINER

Department of Epidemiology and Preventive Medicine, School of Public Health and Preventive Medicine, Monash University, Melbourne, Australia

Abstract

Social media has enabled information, communication and reach for health professionals. There are clear benefits to patients and consumers when health information is broadcast. But there are unanswered questions on professionalism, education, and the complex mentoring relationship between doctor and student. This personal perspective raises a number of questions: What is online medical professionalism? Can online medical professionalism be taught? Can online medical professionalism be enforced? Is an online presence necessary to achieve the highest level of clinical excellence? Is there evidence that social media is superior to traditional methods of teaching in medical education? Does social media encourage multitasking and impairment of the learning process? Are there downsides to the perfunctory laconic nature of social media? Does social media waste time that is better spent attaining clinical skills?

Introduction

As Faust, seated in his arched, Gothic chamber, begins his great tragedy, he is restless, confused and probably dispirited (von Goethe, 1808/2005). This is clear from his first words 'Scene 1. Night (Faust's Monologue)' sic:

I've studied now Philosophy
And Jurisprudence, Medicine,—
And even, alas! Theology,—
From end to end, with labor keen;
And here, poor fool! with all my lore
I stand, no wiser than before

This is how I feel despite many years devoted to social media and medicine. From the launch of my blog AllergyNet Australia in January 1998, almost certainly the first medical blog in the world, to the posting of over 10,000 tweets in six years, and culminating in a rigorous approach to studying this topic as a PhD student, I, like Faust, remain restless and confused about this topic.

Why?

How can a believer feel this way when Kevin Pho, founder of KevinMD.com, which *Forbes* hails as a 'must-read' blog, and whose opinion pieces appear in multiple traditional and online media sites, says 'We need to show our colleagues the value of social media'? (Pho, 2011).

How can we doubt the value of social media in healthcare when the Mayo Clinic offers social media residencies? (Mayo Clinic, 2014).

How can we disregard widespread advice, such as from the editor of the *Journal of the Kentucky Medical Association* that 'Social media can make you a better doctor'? (Mandrola, 2014).

There is no argument that the Internet is unsurpassed when it comes to information, communication and reach. But is public interaction via digital media, inherent in any definition of social media, necessary in medical practice? I feel that there are problems that the avid proponents of social media must solve. These involve overlapping problems of professionalism, education and tutorialism (Fig. 1).

Professionalism

While professionalism in medical practice is clearly important, I would go so far as to suggest it is the sine qua non of medical practice. But there are unanswered questions about professionalism even without introducing social media as an additional variable.

What is medical professionalism?

Medical professionalism, whether online or not, is impossible to define. Yet everyone seems to know

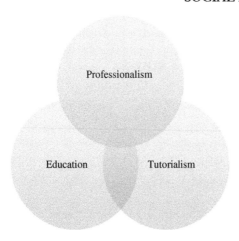

Fig. 1. Overlapping issues of concern in social media and medicine. Tutorialism: A traditional relationship between the doctor as guardian and the student as apprentice where the doctor transfers knowledge, skills and mentorship by ongoing often complex interactions (neologism – see text).

what it is. It is analogous to the definition of pornography that Justice Potter Stewart of the US Supreme Court described in 1964: 'I shall not today attempt further to define the kinds of material I understand to be embraced within that shorthand description [hard-core pornography], and perhaps I could never succeed in intelligibly doing so. But *I know it when I see it*' (Wikipedia, 2014).

The problem of defining professionalism is threefold. Firstly, inherent in assessing professionalism is an ethical construct. Secondly, this assessment varies with the cultural proclivities of the discussants. Finally, there are multiple domains of professionalism. Attempts to define professionalism, such as 'a general standard of all round proficiency and accountability' presuppose a clear understanding of the terms 'general standard', 'proficiency' and 'accountability' (Kerridge et al., 2013).

Transposing clinical professionalism to online professionalism magnifies the opportunity to divert from professionalism however defined. While not in itself an insurmountable block to social media engagement, it nevertheless is a source of anxiety from registration boards down to individual practitioners.

A further problem is the tendency to 'reinvent the wheel' during discussions on professionalism and social media. Whether it is Hippocrates or Osler or Facebook, the guidelines should be the same. But it is not seen that way by many.

For example, a joint initiative of the Australian Medical Association Council of Doctors-in-Training, the New Zealand Medical Association Doctors-in-Training Council, the New Zealand Medical Students' Association and the Australian Medical Students' Association has produced a document called 'Social media and the medical profession' (Mansfield et al., 2011). The advice includes, inter alia, this statement:

Our perceptions and regulations regarding professional behaviour *must evolve to encompass these new forms of media.* (my italics)

I would argue that perceptions and regulations of professionalism, once properly espoused and documented, should be applied universally, in any day and age, and for any circumstance or technology. This is declared, for example, in the Royal Australian and New Zealand College of Psychiatrists Position Statement 'Psychiatry, online presence and social media' (RANZCP, 2012) where, although there are specific allusions to social media behaviour in the document, there is an over-riding clause that clearly states:

they must ensure their social media use and Internet presence upholds the ethical and practice standards required for Fellowship of the College. (RANZCP, 2012)

Others argue that social media is somehow different. After all, it has immediacy and reach and permanency. I cannot accept that a smart, well-educated student who has achieved entry to medical school does not know these properties of social media.

Can medical professionalism be taught?

Many medical schools provide courses in medical professionalism, but there is a strong argument that it cannot be taught, only enforced (see below). Thomas Huddle has argued: 'As attractive as it may be to view professionalism as expertise or as a competence, I will contend that in asking for professionalism, that is, for just, altruistic, conscientious, and compassionate physicians and trainees, medical educators are asking for morality' p. 886 and he concludes 'although medical educators can teach professionalism, especially during internship and residency, we are mistaken to suppose that we can do so as readily as we teach clinical medicine' p. 890 (Huddle, 2005). I find Huddle's arguments persuasive.

The immediate corollary is that online professionalism may be as difficult to teach as clinical professionalism, if not impossible in some students. This will be of concern to many physicians.

Can medical professionalism be enforced?

Here the problem is different. Yes, in principle, rules and regulations are enforceable. But in this case we must admit that maintenance of the same standards on social media is more complex than in real life. Not by behaviour, or definitions, or standards, which are the same in both spheres. But it is more complex because of publicity and reach.

Let me provide an example. In 2014, the Australian Health Practitioner Regulation Agency (AHPRA) attempted to introduce new social media guidelines that included:

> A practitioner must take reasonable steps to have any testimonials associated with their health service or business removed when they become aware of them, even if they appear on a website that is not directly associated and/or under the direct control or administration of that health practitioner. (TressCox, 2014)

The Australian health Twittersphere went into meltdown. Opponents of this proposed regulation, including myself, convinced AHPRA, because of publicity and reach, to modify and effectively reverse it.

While this can be seen as a good outcome in this instance, what if many experienced health professionals saw a proposed legislation as highly desirable, but the public and significant numbers of professionals opposed it. Can an outcome in this instance be democratic? Indeed, should an outcome be democratic?

The concepts of privacy are integral to procuring general agreement in the principles outlined above. Privacy boundaries are clear to physicians who were brought up in the pre-social media era, but are blurred in a significant number of current active users. A cross-sectional survey of the use of Facebook by recent medical graduates found a quarter of the doctors did not use the privacy options, allowing public access to the information they posted (MacDonald et al., 2010). Some of the posts included photographs or descriptions of offensive behaviour, drunkenness, or inappropriate personal information or views. Clearly, growing up with social media seems to produce a perception in a minority of supposedly intelligent and educated health professionals that privacy is in some way a restriction of freedom. I argue that this attitudinal change may be difficult to reverse. But breaches of privacy can certainly be enforced.

Is an online presence necessary to achieve the highest level of clinical excellence?

Clinical excellence, like medical professionalism, is difficult, perhaps impossible to define, yet many professional bodies have adopted criteria for excellence. Indeed, professionalism is usually included as one of the domains of excellence.

The Miller-Coulson Academy (Johns Hopkins Centre for Innovative Medicine, 2014) has developed strong domains with which to judge clinical excellence: communication and interpersonal skills, professionalism and humanism, diagnostic acumen, skilful negotiation of the healthcare system, knowledge, scholarly approach to clinical practice, passion for clinical medicine, and reputation for clinical excellence. An online presence may contribute to any of these domains, especially to communication, but is not essential. Of course, I cannot discount the possibility that, when clinical excellence is analysed in a similar way in the future, an effective social media presence might be considered a marker per se of clinical excellence. Currently, however, there is no evidence that a good virtual doctor is a good real doctor.

Education

Kirkpatrick's four-level model of criteria to assess learning outcomes, as adapted by Praslova, provides a validated tool to study education in higher institutions (Praslova, 2010). Briefly, these criteria are reaction (students' affective reaction to learning), learning (direct measures of learning outcomes), behaviour (evidence that students use knowledge and skills), and results (career success and service to society). Many equate the first criterion (reaction) with success in education. When students are happy, excited, involved, and, critically, 'not bored' by teaching using social media, the teacher might well be satisfied. But the other three criteria must also be fulfilled to determine educational success, and important questions remain to be answered.

Is there evidence that social media is superior to traditional methods of teaching in medical education?

Social media allows access to knowledge. But does it make you think? Is thinking important in clinical practice?

I recently enjoyed watching a lecture by Samuel Gershon, a clinician well-known to readers of this journal (Australian National University, 2010) At the time he was receiving the Curtin Medal for Excellence in Medical Research at the Australian National University on 16 August 2010. He was then the Emeritus Professor of Psychiatry at the University of Pittsburgh. I enjoyed his relaxed presentation of research in Melbourne during the 1950s. He alluded to John Cade's discovery of lithium, and discussed his own collaboration with Edward Troutner of measurement of lithium levels. I pricked up my ears when he revealed that the research was done in the laboratories of Roy Douglas Wright, a brilliant, ambitious and passionate researcher and teacher. I was fortunate to receive lectures from Professor Wright as a second-year medical student in 1967. Wright espoused the Oxford tutorial approach (Oxford Learning Institute, 2014). Today this would be called the inverted or flipped classroom. Several thousand years ago it was a Socratic debate. The flipped classroom is excitedly called a revolution in teaching. It is not.

That is the first problem when analysing social media for teaching – does a change in technology actually mean a different outcome to teaching? Is a YouTube lecture actually intrinsically different from a 'live' lecture? Does online interaction between students actually differ in attaining knowledge and understanding compared to a feisty discussion over beer and pizza? Yes, I understand about communication and reach, but I argue that new technology is not the same as better teaching. We need evidence, not just by a demonstration of better marks, but over a generation of these 'new' doctors.

The first systematic review of social media for medical education analysed 14 studies through September 2011 (Cheston et al., 2013). While most studies were heterogeneous and not of high quality, the authors noted 'it is encouraging to see that several relatively rigorous studies have emerged so early' p. 896 and that 'this systematic review offers a foundation for future research and guidance for incorporating social media tools into medical curricula.' p. 897

My disquiet therefore occurs because, while the academic community slowly collects rigorous data, many online proponents confuse technology with teaching, social media with skills, and access to knowledge with the ability to think.

Does social media encourage multitasking and impairment of the learning process?

Media multitasking is the consumption of more than one item or stream of content at the same time. Heavy media multitaskers are more susceptible to interference from irrelevant environmental stimuli and from irrelevant representations in memory (Ophir et al., 2009). Many studies have examined this and other phenomena. Even when laptops are used solely to take notes, thus not fulfilling the criterion of media multitasking, they may still be impairing learning because their use results in shallower processing (Mueller & Oppenheimer, 2014).

As both a teacher, and recently as a student again, I view the inexorable march to device-driven rather than brain-driven learning with concern. The former results in the inefficient accumulation of facts, the latter promotes analysis and understanding.

Tutorialism

I have used this term for many years but I admit that it is a neologism, albeit I would argue a useful one. The term has appeared in occasional blogs, though

not in the manner in which I use it, and remains officially undefined. A definition would involve concepts of guardianship, protection and teaching, but in a specific medical sense. It might be the consultant and registrar, or the attending and the resident, or the senior consultant and the junior consultant, but the interaction is always the same. It is frank but nurturing, instructive but caring, and is often complex and difficult. I would define tutorialism thus: 'A traditional relationship between the doctor as guardian and the student as apprentice where the doctor transfers knowledge, skills and mentorship by ongoing often complex interactions.' Can social media provide tutorialism? This question does need to be teased out.

Are there downsides to the perfunctory laconic nature of social media?

Information on social media is usually fast and short. This is terrific for letting the world know about an impending disaster. But is speed and brevity conducive to tutorialism? I would argue that it is not.

The social media platforms that could mount a difficult or long argument usually engage in censorship with respect to length. We are told that people get bored with a blog that is over 300–600 words (Bunting, 2014) and the ideal length for a video (with few exceptions) should be 90 s to 3 min (Camp, 2013). Nevertheless, one or two useful facts can be broadcast in that way. I find that useful. But can a complex scenario be discussed in any meaningful way using public comments after the piece? The brevity that is inherent in social media breeds dogmatic and angry responses. In my blog, 80% of comments were insulting, abusive, or motherhood statements, or computer-generated. I finally deleted the ability to comment. You only need to google this problem to realize its extent.

On the other hand, a long and complex blog piece will drive cyber-bullies away but may bore readers silly, because there is no to and fro during the piece, but only comments and replies at the end. Social media is by definition interactive, but not in the tutorialism sense. Tutorialism is a conversation, not a lecture followed by comments and questions. This is a contentious issue, and if this paper were an online blog, the comments section would indeed be long and angry.

Let us examine the common and much-lauded social media activity of live tweeting from a medical conference (Symplur, 2014). Its popularity is engagement. Physicians might feel happy because the snippets that go around the world are comforting in their familiarity. Health consumers might enjoy the headlining fragments about their particular ailment. But this is not tutorialism, and not education. I argue that a physician cannot improve their knowledge from reading a live tweet stream. A physician needs to read papers in detail, discuss issues at length with colleagues, learn or improve skills with practice. I argue that a health consumer cannot improve their well-being by reading a live tweet stream. They are merely a source of insubstantive fragmented news of doubtful significance. Others have aired similar opinions (Skeptical Scalpel, 2014). I would extend this argument to all online discussion groups. They are great for networking, some, such as Reddit, are very good for information, but discussions (as opposed to broadcasts with links) on a platform such as Twitter are generally very unsatisfactory.

In summary, social media, because of brevity and inability to discuss complex issues, certainly does not lend itself to any form of tutorialism, and has limitations with the transfer of knowledge with understanding.

Does social media waste time that is better spent attaining clinical skills?

I raise this point because it is the most frequent criticism I hear from other physicians who are not using social media. A broad debate entitled 'Social media: the way forward or a waste of time for physicians?' is just that – a debate offering two opposing viewpoints (HCSM, 2013) Elsewhere Drummond writes as a comment to his own blog piece on why social media may not be worth it for doctors: 'On your death bed, what do you think your biggest regret will be? ... that you didn't TWEET ENOUGH?' (Drummond, 2012).

There is no replacement for clinical skills. Social media can waste a lot of time. The judicious use of social media is a fine art. I have reduced my volume of social media by 50% in the last 12 months. I see 'waste of time' as a legitimate criticism for excessive interaction. That time is usually better spent in a tutorialism relationship.

Different platforms do complement each other. A tweet can point to a post that can link to a Facebook page. This is useful if broadcasting only. It all depends on why a physician spends time on social media. Multiple platforms promote reach, one platform allows a large amount of interaction, if so desired, and a specialized platform, such as ResearchGate, supports occasional yet effective use. I feel that physicians should be highly selective. I disapprove of those who criticize 'lurkers', a term for those who follow or join but do not interact. Also, those who criticize physicians who are not on social media unsettle me.

Conclusion

What do patients actually want in their physician? Patients want eye contact, partnership, communication, and time (Stone, 2003). I would add reflection not precipitancy, knowledge not guesswork, and skills not ineptness. The jury is still out on whether patients need, rather than want, their physician to be on social media.

As an early adopter, my personal reflection on social media is finely balanced. The benefits of knowledge, communication and reach are clear. But the areas of professionalism, clinical excellence, content, time, distractions and need remain nebulous. And I do not see a role of social media in what I have defined as tutorialism. I admit it may be an age-thing. In my 67th year, I do understand, like Faust 'Tis vain, this empty brooding here' 'Scene 1. Night (Faust's Monologue)' sic, but I am optimistic that some, perhaps not all, of the questions I posed may be answered in the next generation.

Declaration of interest: The author reports no conflicts of interest. The author alone is responsible for the content and writing of the paper.

References

Australian National University. (2010). Prof Samuel Gershon: The psychopharmacological specificity of the lithium ion. Retrieved from http://www.youtube.com/watch?v = JCySrIW-wWw

Bunting, J. (2014). How long should your blog post be? A writer's guide. The Write Practice. Retrieved from http://thewritepractice.com/blog-post-length/

Camp, N. (2013). Online video attention span – How long should a video production be? The Video Effect. Retrieved from http://thevideoeffect.tv/2013/05/08/online-video-attention-span-how-long-should-a-video-production-be/

Cheston, C.C., Flickinger, T.E., & Chisolm, M.S. (2013). Social media use in medical education: A systematic review. *Academic Medicine: Journal of the Association of American Medical Colleges*, 88, 893–901. doi:10.1097/ACM.0b013e31828ffc23

Drummond, D. (2012). Why social media may not be worth it for doctors. *MedPage Today*. Retrieved from http://www.kevinmd.com/blog/2012/04/social-media-worth-doctors.html

HCSM. (2013). Social media: The way forward or a waste of time for physicians? Health Care Social Media Monitor on WordPress.com. Retrieved from http://hcsmmonitor.com/2013/12/20/social-media-the-way-forward-or-a-waste-of-time-for-physicians/

Huddle, T.S. (2005). Viewpoint: Teaching professionalism: Is medical morality a competency? *Academic Medicine : Journal of the Association of American Medical Colleges*, 80, 885–891. doi:10.1097/00001888-200510000-00002

Johns Hopkins Centre for Innovative Medicine. (2014). The Miller-Coulson Academy of Clinical Excellence. Johns Hopkins Medicine. Retrieved 12 October 2014 from http://www.hopkinsmedicine.org/innovative/signature_programs/academy_of_clinical_excellence/

Kerridge, I., Lowe, M., & Stewart, C. (2013). *Ethics and Law for the Health Professions* (4th ed., pp. 161–162). Annandale, NSW: The Federation Press.

MacDonald, J., Sohn, S., & Ellis, P. (2010). Privacy, professionalism and Facebook: A dilemma for young doctors. *Medical Education*, 44, 805–813. doi:10.1111/j.1365-2923.2010.03720.x

Mandrola, J.M. (2014). Dr. John M. Doctors and social media – It's time to embrace change. Dr. John M blog. Retrieved from http://www.drjohnm.org/2014/02/doctors-and-social-media-its-time-to-embrace-change/

Mansfield, S.J., Morrison, S.G., Stephens, H.O., Bonning, M.A., Wang, S.-H., Withers, A.H.J., ... Perry, A.W. (2011). Social media and the medical profession. *Medical Journal of Australia, 194,* 642–644. Retrieved from https://www.mja.com.au/journal/2011/194/12/social-media-and-medical-profession

Mayo Clinic. (2014). Social media residency. *Social Media Health Network.* Retrieved 12 October 2014, from http://network.socialmedia.mayoclinic.org/social-media-residency/

Mueller, P.A., & Oppenheimer, D.M. (2014). The pen is mightier than the keyboard: Advantages of longhand over laptop note taking. *Psychological Science, 25,* 1159–1168. doi:10.1177/0956797614524581

Ophir, E., Nass, C., & Wagner, A.D. (2009). Cognitive control in media multitaskers. *Proceedings of the National Academy of Sciences of the United States of America, 106,* 15583–15587. doi:10.1073/pnas.0903620106

Oxford Learning Institute. (2014). Tutorial teaching. Oxford University. Retrieved 12 October 2014, from https://www.learning.ox.ac.uk/support/teaching/resources/teaching/

Pho, K. (2011). Show doctors the value when it comes to social media and EMRS. Retrieved from http://www.kevinmd.com/blog/2011/12/show-doctors-social-media-emrs.html

Praslova, L. (2010). Adaptation of Kirkpatrick's four level model of training criteria to assessment of learning outcomes and program evaluation in higher education. *Educational Assessment, Evaluation and Accountability, 22,* 215–225. doi:10.1007/s11092-010-9098-7

RANZCP. (2012). Position Statement 75. Psychiatry, online presence and social media. Royal Australian and New Zealand College of Psychiatrists. Retrieved from https://www.ranzcp.org/Files/Resources/College_Statements/Position_Statements/75-Psychiatry,-online-presence-and-social-media-GC.aspx

Ruiz, R. (2009). Must-read health blogs. *Forbes.* Retrieved from http://www.forbes.com/2009/10/07/best-health-blogs-lifestyle-health-blogs-health-information.html

Skeptical Scalpel. (2014). The problem with live tweeting medical conferences. *MedPage Today.* Retrieved from http://www.kevinmd.com/blog/2014/06/problem-live-tweeting-medical-conferences.html

Stone, M. (2003). What patients want from their doctors. *BMJ, 326*(7402), 1294. doi:10.1136/bmj.326.7402.1283-b

Symplur. (2014). Healthcare conferences. Retrieved 12 October 2014 from http://www.symplur.com/healthcare-hashtags/conferences/

TressCox (2014). AHPRA updates the rules: Testimonials and social media are in the regulator's sights. TressCox Lawyers. Retrieved from http://www.tresscox.com.au/resources/resource.asp?id = 1474#.VDn2MlY9KCQ

von Goethe, J.W. (1808/2005). *Faust.* Project Gutenberg. Retrieved 12 October 2014 from http://www.gutenberg.org/files/14591/14591-h/14591-h.htm

Wikipedia. (2014). I know it when I see it. Retrieved 12 October 2014 from http://en.wikipedia.org/wiki/I_know_it_when_I_see_it

Personal reflections on exploring social media in medicine

BRENT THOMA

Department of Emergency Medicine, University of Saskatchewan, Saskatoon, Saskatchewan, Canada

Abstract

Social media is difficult to explain to a physician who has never used it. The medical literature on its pitfalls and abuses has overshadowed its positive applications and made many physicians wary of it. While I was initially reluctant to develop my own presence on social media, since embracing it as a tool for teaching and learning I have developed a different perspective. I see it as a tool that can be used positively or negatively. Much like a megaphone, it can amplify our voice so that the impact of our work can extend beyond the borders of our institutions and countries. Aided by the guidance and support of mentors who used social media before and alongside me, it has helped me to become a more competent, professional, engaged, and impactful physician. Within this article I will share my story to illustrate the many ways that social media can be used to enhance the profession of medicine.

Introduction

I have difficulty explaining the benefits of social media to physicians who have never used it. When they find out I tweet, their initial reactions often convey confusion about why I would waste my time or contain jokes about celebrities I have never heard of. It does not help that the dialogue within the medical literature initially focused on social media's pitfalls and potential for abuse (Farnan et al., 2008; Greysen et al., 2010; Shore et al., 2011; Snyder, 2011). My explorations of social media have led me to view it differently. I see it as a tool. Just as a scalpel can be viewed both as a weapon and an instrument of healing, social media can be thought of as an amplifier that raises the volume on a message, be it good or bad.

At first I did not 'get' social media. I was introduced to its professional uses by my assistant program director, Nadim Lalani, as a junior resident. He raved about the discussions that he was having online and this 'blog' called 'Life in the Fast Lane'. I figured that was just another one of his quirks (he also has an infatuation with fashion and an encyclopaedic knowledge of pop culture). While I began using these resources regularly, I never dreamed that 'interactive websites' would become such a huge part of my professional world. And yet, I now wonder what life would be like had I never started my blog or signed in to Twitter.

My take on social media use in medicine began to shift during my third year of residency shortly after I completed my speciality's annual Canadian in-training exam. My results were compared with residents across the country and I was falling behind in the basic aspects of emergency medicine (e.g. geriatrics, paediatrics, and dermatology). My program director, Rob Woods, asked how I thought I could rectify that and I laughed while saying 'Maybe I'll start writing one of those blogs – I'll call it "BoringEM"!'

While I was not serious at the time, the more that I thought about it the more it made sense. The depth and breadth of knowledge required to regularly create learning resources on these topics would ensure that I addressed a deficiency in my knowledge base. Additionally, most of the online resources in emergency medicine that were available online at the time focused on the high adrenaline and cutting-edge aspects of emergency medicine (e.g. airway management and ultrasound) and had likely contributed to my understanding of these areas. Writing a blog aimed at the more common aspects of emergency medicine practice would both fill a niche and help me to focus my learning on these very important topics.

A week later, BoringEM was born and I began to explore social media in earnest. This reflection tells the story of how I began using it to learn and ended up a more professional physician with a global community of practice (Hochradel, 2013; Wenger, 1990). I hope those reading this story will consider how they can benefit from the use of these exceptional tools.

How has social media affected me?

Education

My initial objective when I began using social media was to learn by creating summaries of my readings that I would post on the new BoringEM blog. From an educational standpoint this strategy made sense. Composing a blog post requires the analysis, application, and evaluation of knowledge – some of the most effective levels of Bloom's taxonomy of learning (Anderson et al., 2001). Blogging helped to take the passive learning that I was doing while reading textbooks and articles and convert it into a more active and productive process (Michael, 2006). However, I was caught off guard by how much I enjoyed creating resources to help others learn.

Ultimately, it was the interactive aspects of social media that drew me in. The online medical education community embraced my blog and helped it to grow quickly. My first post was on interpreting urinalyses (Thoma, 2012) and caught the attention of Mike Cadogan, an Australian innovator in online medical education and one of the founders of the large 'Life in the Fast Lane' blog. He endorsed my post on Twitter and it received nine comments and 400 views within a few days. BoringEM's focus on providing basic content written in an entertaining, or 'edutaining' (Corona et al., 2013), style found an unfilled niche and I was energized by the ability to contribute to the learning of others. Additionally, having an audience meant that readers frequently left comments with questions, suggestions, or corrections that gave me the opportunity to learn with and from them. Ultimately, these interactions had me writing not because I had to, but because I enjoyed it.

Despite these benefits, posting frequent updates to the blog on a resident schedule posed a substantial challenge. Within a year I began looking for others interested in contributing as authors. Teresa Chan, a new assistant professor of emergency medicine and fellow Canadian, was one of the first people to become a regular contributor and was quickly hooked by blogging's potential as an education platform. She developed and implemented a broader vision for the platform that fostered the development of learners while increasing the blog's sustainability.

The largest part of this vision was a mentored peer and expert review process to support medical students and residents who write for BoringEM. Prior to the publication of their work it is reviewed by an internal peer reviewer (often another student or resident) for style, flow, and content. Medical student (Eve Purdy) and resident (Sarah Luckett-Gatopolous) editors were recruited to facilitate this process. Reviews from staff physicians are also solicited to ensure accuracy. The goal of these reviews is not to accept or reject submissions, but to improve their credibility and quality. The writers benefit from a forum that provides frequent feedback on their writing, critical thinking, and literature appraisal skills, while the junior editors develop comfort with the production and assessment of written submissions. We believe that this supportive editorial structure will not only improve our blog's sustainability but, if adopted more broadly, could foster the next generation of academic writers and editors.

Professionalism

Much of the academic literature published in medical journals on social media has focused on its danger to physicians (Cunningham, 2014; DeCamp, 2012; Greysen et al., 2010; Moses et al., 2014; Shore et al., 2011; Snyder, 2011). While its positive applications for teaching (Cheston et al., 2013), educators (Forgie et al., 2013; Kind et al., 2014), clinicians (Batt-Rawden et al., 2014), and academics (Chu et al., 2010) have also been described, as a medical student and resident I found that these messages were overshadowed by negative articles, presentations, and communications. For example, during the annual residency match many of my classmates deleted or obscured their social media profiles because they had heard that residency programs will be looking online for red flags (Cain et al., 2010). My experience with social media has been much more consistent with the positive literature.

As a medical student I made a mistake that involved a more traditional academic medium. I submitted a description of one of my early clinical experiences (performing a pap smear) that went poorly, to my country's largest family medicine journal (Thoma, 2009). It included several crude jokes, some that were made at the expense of a patient, and many patients and physicians were offended. I regret having written or shared it in any forum. Following its publication multiple letters were written to the editor that describe the controversy (Andres, 2010; Greenberg, 2010; Joo, 2010; Ogle, 2010; Tai, 2010; Thoma, 2010) which was also discussed in newspapers around the world. It was an extremely difficult time for me, both personally and professionally, and I thank those who supported me at the time and the residency program that gave me another chance. As a result of this publication, before starting my blog my online reputation was predominantly negative and I was extremely wary of writing anything for public distribution.

During my first months of blogging I wrote my posts under a pseudonym, fearful that something similar would happen. At the same time, I did my utmost to ensure that my content was highly appropriate, frequently having my posts reviewed by my program directors, other attending physicians at my institution, and occasionally other medical bloggers.

Navigating this early period required an acknowledgement of my limits as a junior physician, the support and guidance of my mentors and residency program, and substantial introspection. When the article on pap smears was brought up several years later I was able to use my blog as a forum to respond appropriately (Thoma, 2013).

Ultimately, social media helped me to find my voice again by allowing me to write in a smaller forum that, while still public, was made safer by knowing that my content had been vetted. While the feedback of my mentors did not result in substantial changes for professionalism reasons, I suspect this was because I had learned from my previous experiences and from the way they modelled professionalism through their own use of social media. I believe that writing a blog regularly and conscientiously while maintaining a public presence on social media has contributed to my development as a professional, rather than inhibiting it.

By fostering a strong online persona I found that I had much more agency over my digital presence. A Google search of my name was not flattering following the publication of my controversial article. However, by having a consistent and professional online presence over a number of years I became defined by this work, rather than that single event. Ultimately, I feel that I was able to use social media to develop and demonstrate professionalism. Similar benefits have been described by others (Kind et al., 2013).

Networking

As both a medical student and a resident I trained at the University of Saskatchewan. It is a small medical school in a sparsely populated Canadian province. My decision to study there was driven first by geography (it is where I grew up) and later by opportunity (I was one of the first residents in a brand new program). While the advantages of attending a small medical school are numerous, the faculty, resources, connections, and alumni network at its disposal are necessarily limited.

As I continued to interact online I began to make friends with other physicians and healthcare professionals. A growing number of the medical bloggers and podcasters believed strongly in sharing resources freely online (Cadogan et al., 2014). They rallied around the hashtag #FOAMed or 'Free Open Access Medical education' on Twitter and supported each other's work (Nickson & Cadogan, 2014). Effectively, they formed a virtual community of practice (Hochradel, 2013; Wenger, 1990) focused on developing educational and technological capacity in online medical education. As an example of the extent to which these strangers would go to help each other, two months after my first post on BoringEM,

Mike Cadogan transitioned my website to a new server and dramatically improved its functionality for free and on his own time.

This was but the first of many times that I received assistance and opportunities as a result of my online engagement. Social media largely eliminated the barriers created by distance and gave me the chance to learn from and work with an international community of exceptional physicians. Many of the papers that I have written over the past year are the result of collaboration with individuals whom I have not met in person and may have never interacted with if it were not for social media.

Scholarship

As my residency progressed I became increasingly interested in a career in academic medicine. Having devoted substantial time and effort to my blog I wondered about its acceptance as a scholarly activity. If I ever had any question that its scholarly value would be doubtful, I received an answer at one of my program research days: during the question period I asked an eminent visiting researcher whether he felt that resources like the ones I was creating had or ever would have scholarly value. His response was succinct and concise: 'No, never.'

Traditionally, educational scholarship has been defined as work that is peer reviewed, publicly disseminated, and can be built upon by others (Canadian Association for Medical Education Advancement of Education Scholarship Working Group, 2012). The knock against social media resources such as blogs and podcasts are their lack of traditional, prepublication peer review. While they may never meet this criteria, signs that social media are being increasingly valued in academia abound. In addition to this issue of the *International Review of Psychiatry*, the journal *Emergency Medicine of Australasia* published a social media theme issue in February 2014, and the Royal College of Physicians and Surgeons of Canada convened a Social Media Summit in 2014 that included a consensus conference on the scholarship of social media.

Research was of little interest to me before I discovered social media. I dutifully conducted my residency-required research project, but got little enjoyment out of it. I was once told that research is not interesting until you find a question that you are excited about. After finding social media and its related educational products (blogs, podcasts, screencasts, and vodcasts) so useful for my own education, I became intrigued by questions exploring how they worked and how we could use them better.

The same social media tools that I sought to study quickly connected me with a group of educational scholars with similar interests. Our initial projects led to the establishment of a research collaborative called MedEdLIFE (Leading Innovations that Foster Educators) to coordinate our growing research agenda. Individually, we had struggled to explore a field that does not fit traditional paradigms of medical education research. However, together we have been able to publish some early papers in this growing field of inquiry (Cadogan et al., 2014; Purdy et al., 2014; Thoma et al., 2014a, 2014b, 2014c).

Impact

While I have been a productive resident, the influence that I have gained through my prominence on social media is disproportional to the contributions that I have made. Traditionally, academics work for years to gain influence and credibility by building a track record of publications and speaking engagements at the local, regional, national, and international level. By sharing my work on the Internet I largely bypassed this traditional career progression. Despite being a resident, my social media presence has led to invitations to speak at international conferences and write editorials for journals both within and outside of my speciality.

As this anecdote demonstrates, impact is perhaps the construct that has been most flipped on its head by the growing influence of social media. The appropriateness of this change has rightly been questioned, with one researcher even defining a 'Kardashian Index,' named for the family famous for being famous, to quantify the extent to which an academic's online influence outweighs their contributions to their field (Cox et al., 2014; Hall, 2014). However, academics should realize that this tongue-in-cheek publication demonstrates that if they are not online, opportunities may be offered to their colleagues who are otherwise less established.

The field of altmetrics provides a more legitimate assessment of this phenomenon. Altmetrics, also known as 'alternative metrics' or 'article-level metrics,' consist of a variety of measures of online dissemination (e.g. the frequency that an article is read, saved on reference managers, or discussed in the media, blogs, or social media). With the support of a growing body of literature (Priem, 2013; Roemer & Borchadt, 2012; Thelwall et al., 2013), altmetrics are becoming recognized measures of the impact of individual publications and are being incorporated into the websites of many recognized journals (e.g. *Nature*, Wiley Journals, Cambridge Journals) and repositories (e.g. Elsevier ScienceDirect). The altmetrics for my research have increased tremendously because I am able to disseminate it using social media. In the future, these impact metrics may also be considered for grant and promotion applications in the same way that citations are now (Kwok, 2013; Piwowar, 2013).

Practice

Social media helps to keep me up to date on practice-changing literature. For example, within a week of the publication of a study that largely changed the use of therapeutic hypothermia following cardiac arrest (Nielsen et al., 2013), it was discussed on 17 blogs and podcasts that I follow (Thoma et al., 2014d). As a result of my social media engagement, I quickly had knowledge of this trial and absorbed multiple perspectives on its implications for my practice.

I have been introduced to a number of diverse resources through social media. I believe this is important because these less conventional resources often provide alternative perspectives on the published literature. For example, they include strong, evidence-based arguments against the use of thrombolytics in acute ischaemic stroke (Newman, 2013) that run counter to the guidelines of many specialist societies (Jauch et al., 2013). The correct balance between novel and traditional resources has not yet been established; however, I strongly believe that my practice and patients benefit from the knowledge that I gain by absorbing and contributing to this dialogue.

Conclusion

I never thought social media was for me, but it has helped me to become a more competent, professional, engaged, and impactful physician. We must not think of it as good or evil, but a tool whose values are determined by the one who wields it. For our junior colleagues to benefit from the positive aspects of social media in the way that I have we must use it alongside them, modelling appropriate behaviour while at the same time supporting their professional development. I hope that this reflection on social media in medicine will prompt further discussion and research on the merits of its use by physicians.

Acknowledgements

The author would like to acknowledge Teresa Chan and Rob Woods for providing feedback on this manuscript.

Declaration of interest: The author reports no conflicts of interest. Brent Thoma was responsible for the conception, design, analysis, interpretation, drafting, revision, and final content of the submitted article.

References

Anderson, L.W., Krathwohl, D.R., Airasian, P.W., Cruikshank, K.A., Mayer, R.E., Pintrich, P.R., ... Wittrock, M.C. (2001). *A Taxonomy for learning, teaching, and assessing: A revision of*

Bloom's taxonomy of educational objectives (abridged). White Plains, NY: Longman.

Andres, D.E. (2010). The other side of the speculum debate. *Canadian Family Physician, 56,* 221. Retrieved from http://www.cfp.ca/content/55/11/1112.short/reply#cfp_el_1065

Batt-Rawden, S., Flickinger, T., Weiner, J., Cheston, C., & Chisolm, M. (2014). The role of social media in clinical excellence. *Clinical Teacher, 11,* 264–269.

Cadogan, M., Thoma, B., Chan, T.M., & Lin, M. (2014). Free Open Access Meducation (FOAM): The rise of emergency medicine and critical care blogs and podcasts (2002–2013). *Emergency Medicine Journal, 31,* e76–e77. doi:10.1136/emermed-2013-203502

Cain, J., Scott, D.R., & Smith, K. (2010). Use of social media by residency program directors for resident selection. *American Journal of Health-System Pharmacy, 67*(19), 1635–1639. doi:10.2146/ajhp090658

Canadian Association for Medical Education Advancement of Education Scholarship Working Group. (2012). *'Toward a Common Understanding' Advancing Educational Scholarship for Clinical Faculty in Canadian Medical Schools.* Ottawa, ON: Canadian Association for Medical Education.

Cheston, C.C., Flickinger, T.E., & Chisolm, M.S. (2013). Social media use in medical education: A systematic review. *Academic Medicine, 88*(6), 893–901. doi:10.1097/ACM.0b013e31828ffc23

Chu, L.F., Zamora, A.K., Young, C.A., Kurup, V., & Macario, A. (2010). The role of social networking applications in the medical academic environment. *International Anesthesiology Clinics, 48*(3), 61–82.

Corona, F., Cozzarelli, C., Palumbo, C., & Sibilio, M. (2013). Information technology and edutainment: Education and entertainment in the age of interactivity. *International Journal of Digital Literacy and Digital Competence, 4*(1), 12–18. doi:10.4018/jdldc.2013010102

Cox, B., Myers, P.Z., Wiseman, R., Krauss, L.M., Greene, B., & Carroll, S.M. (2014). Who are the science stars of Twitter? *Science, 345*(6203), 1440–1441.

Cunningham, A. (2014). Social media and medical professionalism. *Medical Education, 48*(2), 110–2. doi:10.1111/medu.12404

DeCamp, M. (2012). Social media and medical professionalism. *Archives of Internal Medicine, 172*(18), 1418–1419. doi:10.1001/archinternmed.2012

Farnan, J.M., Paro, J.A, Higa, J., Edelson, J., & Arora, V.M. (2008). The YouTube generation: implications for medical professionalism. *Perspectives in Biology and Medicine, 51*(4), 517–24. doi:10.1353/pbm.0.0048

Forgie, S.E., Duff, J.P., & Ross, S. (2013). Twelve tips for using Twitter as a learning tool in medical education. *Medical Teacher, 35,* 8–14. doi:10.3109/0142159X.2012.746448

Greenberg, G.R. (2010). A lesson in patient-centred interviewing. *Canadian Family Physician, 56,* 17.

Greysen, S.R., Kind, T., & Chretien, K.C. (2010). Online professionalism and the mirror of social media. *Journal of General Internal Medicine, 25*(11), 1227–1229. doi:10.1007/s11606-010-1447-1

Hall, N. (2014). The Kardashian index: A measure of discrepant social media profile for scientists. *Genome Biology, 15*(7), 424. doi:10.1186/s13059-014-0424-0

Hochradel, C.B. (2013). *Communities of Practice.* University of Massachusetts. Retrieved from http://scholarworks.umb.edu/cgi/viewcontent.cgi?article = 1006 & context = instruction_capstone

Jauch, E.C., Saver, J.L., Adams, H.P., Bruno, A., Connors, J.J.B., Demaerschalk, B.M., ... Yonas, H. (2013). Guidelines for the early management of patients with acute ischemic stroke: A guideline for healthcare professionals from the American Heart Association/American Stroke Association. *Stroke, 44*(3), 870–947. doi:10.1161/STR.0b013e318284056a

Joo, P. (2010). Give him a break! *Canadian Family Physician.* Retrieved from http://www.cfp.ca/content/55/11/1112.short/reply#cfp_el_1065

Kind, T., Patel, P.D., & Lie, D.A. (2013). Opting in to online professionalism: Social media and pediatrics. *Pediatrics, 132*(5), 792–5. doi:10.1542/peds.2013-2521

Kind, T., Patel, P.D., Lie, D., & Chretien, K.C. (2014). Twelve tips for using social media as a medical educator. *Medical Teacher, 36*(4), 284–290. doi:10.3109/0142159X.2013.852167

Kwok, R. (2013). Altmetrics make their mark. *Nature, 500,* 491–493. doi:10.1038/nj7463-491a

Michael, J. (2006). Where's the evidence that active learning works? *Advances in Physiology Education, 30*(4), 159–167. doi:10.1152/advan.00053.2006

Moses, R.E., McNeese, L.G., Feld, L.D., & Feld, A.D. (2014). Social media in the health-care setting: Benefits but also a minefield of compliance and other legal issues. *American Journal of Gastroenterology, 109*(8), 1128–32. doi:10.1038/ajg.2014.67

Newman, D. (2013). Thrombolytics for acute ischemic stroke. Retrieved December 09, 2014, from http://www.thennt.com/nnt/thrombolytics-for-stroke/

Nickson, C.P., & Cadogan, M.D. (2014). Free Open Access Medical education (FOAM) for the emergency physician. *Emergency Medicine Australasia, 26,* 76–83. doi:10.1111/1742-6723.12191

Nielsen, N., Wetterslev, J., Cronberg, T., Erlinge, D., Gasche, Y., Hassager, C., ... Friberg, H. (2013). Targeted temperature management at 33°C versus 36°C after cardiac arrest. *New England Journal of Medicine, 369*(23), 2197–2206. doi:10.1056/NEJMoa1310519

Ogle, K.D. (2010). Printing error? *Canadian Family Physician, 56,* 17.

Piwowar, H. (2013). Value all research products. *Nature, 493*(10), 159. doi:10.1038/493159a

Priem, J. (2013). Beyond the paper. *Nature, 495,* 437–440. doi:10.1038/495437a

Purdy, E., Thoma, B., Bednarczyk, J., Migneault, D., & Sherbino, J. (2014). The use of free online educational resources by Canadian emergency medicine residents and program directors. *Canadian Journal of Emergency Medicine, 17*(2). doi:10.1017/cem.2014.73

Roemer, R.C., & Borchadt, R. (2012). From bibliometrics to altmetrics: A changing scholarly landscape. *College and Research Libraries,* (November), 596–601.

Shore, R., Halsey, J., Shah, K., Crigger, B.-J., & Douglas, S.P. (2011). Report of the AMA Council on Ethical and Judicial Affairs: Professionalism in the use of social media. *Journal of Clinical Ethics, 22*(2), 165–172. Retrieved from http://europepmc.org/abstract/MED/21837888

Snyder, L. (2011). Online professionalism: Social media, social contracts, trust, and medicine. *Journal of Clinical Ethics, 22*(2), 173–175. Retrieved from http://europepmc.org/abstract/MED/21837889

Tai, C. (2010). Concerns about process. *Canadian Family Physician, 56,* 17.

Thelwall, M., Haustein, S., Larivière, V., & Sugimoto, C.R. (2013). Do altmetrics work? Twitter and ten other social web services. *PloS One, 8*(5), e64841. doi:10.1371/journal.pone.0064841

Thoma, B. (2009). The other side of the speculum. *Canadian Family Physician, 55*(11), 1112.

Thoma, B. (2010). Lessons learned. *Canadian Family Physician, 56*(2), 134.

Thoma, B. (2012). Urinalysis voodoo. Retrieved December 06, 2014, from http://boringem.org/2012/12/12/urinalysis-voodoo/

Thoma, B. (2013). Professionalism and I: A controversial publication. Retrieved December 09, 2014, from http://boringem.org/2013/03/05/professionalism-and-i/

Thoma, B., Chan, T., Benitez, J., & Lin, M. (2014a). Educational scholarship in the digital age: A scoping review and analysis of scholarly products. *Winnower, 2,* e14827.77297. doi:10.15200/winn.141827.77297

Thoma, B., Chan, T.M., Desouza, N., & Lin, M. (2014b). Implementing peer review at an emergency Mmdicine blog: Bridging the gap between educators and clinical experts. *Canadian Journal of Emergency Medicine, 16,* 1–4.

Thoma, B., Joshi, N., Trueger, N.S., Chan, T.M., & Lin, M. (2014c). Five strategies to effectively use online resources in emergency medicine. *Annals of Emergency Medicine, 64*(4), 392–395. doi:10.1016/j.annemergmed.2014.05.029

Thoma, B., Rolston, D., & Lin, M. (2014d). Global emergency medicine journal club: Social media responses to the March 2014 Annals of Emergency Medicine journal club on targeted temperature management. *Annals of Emergency Medicine, 64*(2), 207–212. doi:10.1016/j.annemergmed.2014.06.003

Wenger, E. (1990). *Communities of Practice: Learning, Meaning, and Identity.* Cambridge, UK: Cambridge University Press.

My three shrinks: Personal stories of social media exploration

STEVE DAVISS[1], ANNETTE HANSON[2] & DINAH MILLER[3]

[1]*Department of Psychiatry, University of Maryland School of Medicine, Baltimore,* [2]*Department of Forensic Psychiatry, University of Maryland, Baltimore,* [3]*Department of Psychiatry, Johns Hopkins University, Baltimore, Maryland, USA*

Abstract

Three psychiatrist authors illustrate the impact of social media on their professional lives by reflecting on personal stories about their experiences with social media. They reflect on their experiences with listservs, chat rooms, online forums, blogs, podcasts, and other interactive media, while recounting actual stories involving those media. The impact of social media on professional advocacy across broad populations is addressed. In addition, the use of social media in educating psychiatric trainees and informing forensic evaluations is discussed. Finally, social media as a tool for enhancing consumer advocacy and addressing controversial patient safety procedures in emergency settings is discussed.

Introduction

How can social media be used to educate others about the profession of psychiatry and advocate for changes needed? How can it be used to enhance psychiatric training? Can psychiatrists effectively advocate for improvements in patient care?

These are the questions that these three psychiatrist authors illustrate with personal stories about their experiences with social media. The three of them have together maintained a blog since 2006, produced over 65 audio podcasts, written a book about psychiatry for the lay audience, and participated in other forms of social media over the years. They are often referred to as the 'Shrink Rap docs' due to their blog of the same name. They can be reached at mythreeshrinks@gmail.com.

Steve Daviss, a psychosomatic psychiatrist and informatician, tells the story of how he first got involved in social media in 1993 with a schizophrenia listserv, then later chat rooms, blogs, and podcasts. The impact on professional advocacy across broad populations is discussed. Annette Hanson, a forensic psychiatrist and educator, tells her story of how she employs social media to educate trainees, inform forensic evaluations, and stay informed. Dinah Miller, a psychotherapist and author, tells her story of learning through social media about a distressing harmful procedure applied during the hospitalization process, employing social media to survey others' experiences, and then using social media to begin a broad dialogue and advocate for change.

Using social media to advocate for the profession

Steve Daviss

Letter to my malpractice carrier in 2001, protesting their requirement that I cease participating in the dominant social media of the times – chat rooms:

> ... Despite the above information, PRMS has apparently taken a policy that insured psychiatrists would have their coverage dropped if there is evidence that they spend any amount of time (even twelve hours per year) teaching or providing medical educational information in an **online chat room setting**

> As of October 1, 2001, I have ceased to provide such information ... I remain hopeful that PRMS – which is endorsed by the American Psychiatric Association, is thought to be the most progressive insurer for psychiatrists, and considered the Cadillac of coverage – will review this unfortunate policy and determine a more considered and acceptable policy that does not 'gag' its members from speaking about medical issues in online chat rooms.

It was late 1993 after beginning a schizophrenia research fellowship at the Maryland Psychiatric Research Center that I launched my first experiment in social media (no one called it that back then).

Because of my own personal connection with schizophrenia (multiple affected relatives), I had become interested in educating patients, family members, and the general public about ongoing research in schizophrenia and the role that psychiatrists and other mental health professionals play in treatment.

It was also in 1993 that a new communication medium called the 'Internet' was beginning to take off. Gopher (as in 'gopher://') was the then popular Internet protocol used to access documents on servers. Using gopher, I discovered listserv software, which ran on servers that one could subscribe to by adding your email address to a particular listserv topic so that you could participate in a global discussion of that topic. I combed through the listserv servers that I could find and could not find a listserv dedicated to the topic of schizophrenia. So I created one, called SCHIZ-L (Daviss, 1994).

SCHIZ-L quickly became a popular listserv for family members, researchers, clinicians, and patients to connect to and discuss issues related to schizophrenia. Talking directly with each other helped reduce stigma and misunderstandings that people had about the disease, about psychiatrists, and about the profession. After learning so much about the mental health resources available on the Internet, it was through gopher servers that I published *An Internet Primer for Mental Health Professionals* (Daviss,?) where I included SCHIZ-L as one of the many online resources and educated my colleagues about this thing called the Internet. In 1995, when I passed SCHIZ-L on to someone else to manage, we had several hundred participants on SCHIZ-L, and I was convinced that this was an amazing new communication medium that empowered anyone who could access it.

A few years later, America Online (AOL) was the main way many people accessed the Internet, using dial-up modems to send email, browse AOL's walled garden of content, and participate in chat rooms. These chat rooms often had specific topics, rules of engagement, and moderators to maintain some level of order (Gitlow, 2001).

Stuart Gitlow and three friends started a company called Healant that provided online resources via AOL that focused on alternative medicine, substance abuse, and depression. The Depression Information Forum (DIF) was sponsored by Pfizer and provided unbiased information on depression and other mood disorders, including symptoms, diagnosis, differential diagnosis, and treatment. There were also several scheduled chat rooms focusing on depression, known as DIF Chats, that occurred throughout the week.

Stu and I were in the same residency class, so he asked me if I was interested in hosting a weekly 'Ask the Doctor' DIF Chat. I agreed, and in late 1997 or early 1998, I was the Sunday night DIF Chat doctor until I stopped it in late 2001. This was a great experience, one where I helped to educate and support a lot of people who were affected by depression in some way. This was my second experience with what is now called 'social media.' As with SCHIZ-L, I learned that people with different perspectives – patients, clinicians, researchers, family members, policy-makers, educators – could talk openly about their experiences, their beliefs, their biases, and could have frank, reasonable conversations. They could see beyond the stigmas and stereotypes and talk with the 'people', not the 'labels.' The Healant team did a wonderful job facilitating this type of education and support on AOL.

Then, the dot-com crash hit, eventually taking Healant along with it. Just before that happened my malpractice insurer sent out a survey asking, among many other things, about our 'Internet activities.' I described my role in the AOL DIF Chat, making it clear that I did not give out any medical advice, did not make treatment recommendations, and was careful to word all my communications (based on Healant's training) as educational information. They asked for an example, and I sent them a transcript of one chat. They informed me that if I continued to do this they would cancel my malpractice insurance due to the 'undefined liability risk.' They made it clear that their concerns were not due to inside information about risks, but rather that the risks were unknown.

After some protest and attempts to rally the APA for support, I sent a letter that began:

The purpose of this letter is to amend my application for malpractice liability insurance to reflect the fact that I no longer provide educational information about depression and its treatment in a chat room in the Depression Information Forum (DIF) on America Online (AOL).

Fast-forward to 2006, when Dinah Miller, my former medical director at a community mental health clinic, tells me she doesn't really know what it is, but she would like to start a blog 'for psychiatrists, by psychiatrists.' Along with her friend, Anne Hanson, a forensic psychiatrist, the three of us started the Shrink Rap blog using Google's Blogger platform (http://psychiatrist-blog.blogspot.com). While the noun 'shrink' may have a pejorative connotation, we have also found it to be used as an endearing and approachable lay term; when used as a self-reference by psychiatrists, it seems to have a disarming effect that defuses the power relationship between psychiatrist and patient.

Blogging as a form of social media was prevalent by then, though it had the undeserved reputation of being a wasteful form of public navel-gazing (Lenhart & Fox, 2006). Because anyone with access could start a blog, many of them were little more than public diaries filled with daily entries of one's life. But there were also many blogs that focused on topics of interest, both narrow and wide, garnering significant amounts of discussion in the comments section. Healthcare quickly became a popular topic for bloggers, inspiring the first cabinet-level blogger in US history, Secretary of Health Michael Leavitt, to answer the question of whether he thought blogs were going to be a significant part of public policy in government in the future, with the response, 'Absolutely!' (http://en.wikipedia.org/wiki/Mike_Leavitt). This was the third time in 10 years that I had been involved in social media that helps advocate to the public the role that mental health professionals play – first by listserv, then by chat room, then by blog.

An interesting observation relates to anonymity in social media. Early on in the form of social media, it was common to use one's real name. During the explosion of chat rooms and blogs, there seemed to be a greater tendency to use 'screen names' and other pseudonyms to disguise one's identity. With more anonymity came a greater degree of incivility, with an increase in flaming (vitriolic ad hominem attacks) and trolling (intentional inflammatory remarks designed to invoke outrage) behaviours. In healthcare particularly, medical blogs were often anonymous, possibly due to the uncertain risk involved. With malpractice insurers pressuring us to avoid using the Internet at all, it is no wonder that many of us used pseudonyms. The dramatic unmasking of the paediatrician blogger, Robert Lindeman or 'Flea', in 2007 (Saltzman, 2007), presaged the relaxation of concerns about revealing one's identity, as we as a society began to accept the loss of anonymity with the modern Internet. There have since been recommendations on standards for professionalism in social media (DeJong, 2012; Fenwick, 2014; Greysen et al., 2010).

We soon expanded to an auditory form of social media, the podcast. We produced over 65 episodes of our podcast, *My Three Shrinks*, available at mythreeshrinks.com and on iTunes in the Medicine category (https://itunes.apple.com/us/podcast/my-three-shrinks/id207838516). Using humour and humility we were able to engage people and connect with them as people, not as stereotypes. We have slowed down over the past couple years, mostly due to the time challenges of producing a pro bono podcast in one's spare time. We even ventured into traditional media with our book, *Shrink Rap: Three Psychiatrists Explain Their Work* (Miller et al., 2011).

To illustrate the value to professional advocacy of participating in these forms of social media, consider these reviews of our podcast posted to iTunes:

I really like this podcast. I think the reason is that it is a wonderful blend of information and humor. It makes psychotherapy very understandable and shrinks very human, showing psychotherapy as an art, a science and a business ... From these podcasts, you learn a little bit about what's new in psychotherapy and what it's like to practice in today's environment, the joys, the challenges, the pitfalls, the irritants and the rewards. It's a little like getting to listen at the keyhole as the three psychiatrists discuss big and little issues in psychiatry. (mazola)

If you have any interest in the realm of psychiatry then you must listen to this podcast. Dinah, ClinkShrink and Roy do a wonderful job of presenting psychiatric issues in layman's terms that are both easy to understand and hilarious to listen to. Issues they discuss vary from psychiatrists in film and TV to mental health issues that range from depression to identity disorders. It's like going to med school, minus all the studying plus a whole lot cheaper. (ravendancer)

This is really a good show for us lay folks, I really enjoy the banter. Very informative and not a chore to listen to. Please keep up the good work. (tyski1)

We have since used additional forms of social media, including Facebook, Twitter (@shrinkraproy, @HITshrink, @shrinkrapdinah, @clinkshrink), Google+, and Pinterest. All of these tend to serve the purpose of broadening our discussion of medical and mental health issues with a larger, more lay, audience. This deeper connection with people serves to help others see us as people, not just 'psychiatrists' or 'psychologists.' This helps to reduce the negative impact that traditional media (movies, TV, books) have had by representing mental health professionals with stigmatizing qualities. Making these ongoing efforts via social media in an open and engaging way is an important part of advocating for our profession so that others understand us better.

Social media in medical education

Annette Hanson

Steve Daviss's pioneering experience with a discussion board and a listserv served as a forerunner to my experience using social media in medical education. While he used the technology to educate the general public about psychiatric issues, I use social media in my role as a forensic psychiatry training director. Social media content is a unique and valuable addition to my arsenal of teaching tools. Prior to the invention of Facebook, Twitter, YouTube, podcasts, and blogs, medical education was confined to the patient bedside and limited to the one-on-one mentorship of the particular faculty member assigned to that team, at that particular institution. The challenge of a medical educator, and for me as a programme director, is to ensure that each student receives a consistent learning experience and is able to master a uniform curriculum in spite of any differences in training sites or on-site supervision.

Today's medical residents are also more inclined to expect immediate access to digital information. Some bricks-and-mortar health sciences libraries have started to reduce their print subscriptions and have begun converting their holdings to all-electronic formats. As a training director I realized I needed to adapt my teaching style to the demands of my students' schedules, and to provide the information my residents need when and where it is needed. Since training in forensic psychiatry may take place in a hospital, a jail, a prison, or a court clinic, medical education in my subspeciality is not confined to the patient bedside or to a classroom with predefined hours.

Our blog, Shrink Rap, became a place for me to try out ideas and test them with a global audience of colleagues. It was also a place to store and curate information gleaned at conferences and seminars; a quick Google search of the blog could pull up notes from a lecture I vaguely recalled hearing at a conference years before. Those notes tracked the evolution of my thinking about various topics over time, and became the foundation for later papers and columns.

After the blog came Twitter. Some of the early people I followed were journalists who wrote about legal affairs and also a local crime reporter. I was able to hear about newly decided US Supreme Court cases and class action suits pertinent to forensic practice and correctional health care. On a local level, during our state's general assembly my students were able to follow testimony about proposed mental health legislation through a colleague who live-tweeted the event.

Lastly, my Pinterest account has become a convenient place to store 'pins' of forensic reference material and multimedia links. I admit that I may have the most bizarre Pinterest board on the Internet. A quick perusal of my 'pins' turns up content related to facts associated with the killing of elderly wives, articles related to malingered insanity, a first-person account of infanticide, a story about a lawsuit filed by a prison inmate seeking gender reassignment surgery, a list of prison slang, drug court outcome studies, and a cheat sheet listing biographies of all nine US Supreme Court justices.

As inhibitions about the use of social media dropped among physicians, I was pleased to see other respected forensic psychiatrists tweeting out links to news, conferences, and newly published academic papers. In turn, I retweeted and forwarded this information to my students. Social media allowed access to academicians and resources my students would otherwise have no contact with. Similarly, YouTube was a surprising source of training materials. I found videotaped lectures by law professors across the country related to confessions, the role of neuroscience in the legal determination of sanity, and a 3-h course about the use of sex offender risk assessment instruments taught by a nationally renowned expert in these assessments.

Forensic psychiatry involves training in the evaluation of criminal defendants in order to determine legal sanity. Social media content is increasingly part of this process, given the real-time data that it provides about a defendant's mental state at the time of the crime. A student in forensic psychiatry may review Facebook posts, tweets or online videos made by a defendant during the offence. I have adapted my curriculum to include information about digital discovery rules as well as state and federal laws regarding access to electronic communications.

While social media content has been primarily helpful to me as an educator, many of my colleagues have been less enthusiastic about embracing these new tools. The freewheeling and unmoderated style of the Internet feels incompatible with the academician's dispassionate and impartial approach to communication. Many medical educators fear potential repercussions on promotion or professional reputation (Grande et al., 2014). They are concerned that personal and professional identities may become blurred online, and of the risk that embarrassing or overly personal information might be revealed at trial, while on the witness stand during an aggressive cross-examination. 'Has it ever been used against you (in court)?' is a common question I get from colleagues. Clearly they have heard too many horror stories, too many cautionary tales about Facebook posts gone awry, or about people who misinterpret an ineptly worded tweet. Some of these concerns are justified. Unlike traditional media, a misstep online has the potential to spread globally and to be preserved indefinitely.

Nevertheless, the need to maintain a professional public image is not limited to participation in social media. As a medical educator, I hope to train residents to be prepared to step into leadership roles and to guide public policy. This requires the same decorum as one would expect online. Whether testifying in a high profile criminal case in front of traditional media, or blogging about topics relevant to patient care, one needs to be aware that we represent the public face of our profession. What we write, what we tweet, and what we blog will shape the public image of medicine and of the patients we care for.

As Dinah Miller describes next, the use of social media can also be a tool to allow patients to describe their experiences with care – both positive and negative – and to steer our profession in a more humane and compassionate direction.

Social media to advocate for our patients

Dinah Miller

Steve Daviss discussed his personal history using social media to communicate about psychiatry and Annette Hanson further described how she uses social media as a tool for education. I would like to take this one step further and talk about using these forums to understand what our patients are experiencing when they undergo treatment, and how we might use these media to advocate for improvements in care.

While I had seen protestors at the American Psychiatric Association's annual meetings, it was not until we started our Shrink Rap blog that I came to appreciate how distressed some patients could be with the treatment they received during psychiatric crises. In my clinical practice I was not exposed to this; psychiatry is a shortage speciality and people came to outpatient care because they wanted to be there. It was through our readers' comments that I began to hear just how violated some patients felt by a number of aspects of their care.

Social media has been useful to me in many ways over the past 8–9 years, but I am going to focus below on a single example to illustrate how it can help to advocate for our patients.

One reader wrote to complain about being strip searched upon admission to a psychiatric unit. She had been sexually abused earlier in her life, and being searched reactivated distressing memories. She felt that psychiatry should be about healing, not about violation.

Forced treatment was a re-creation of sexual assault for me, which was not life-saving, it was destroying. To be forced to take my clothes off in front of people, to try and hide my body with my arms, to be put in a room with a metal door, to be reduced to pleading and begging, to know my voice meant nothing. It was the same story only with different perpetrators.

I had no idea that patients were searched in this way; no one had ever mentioned it to me. At first, I assumed it was either something specific to this patient, or a uniform policy conducted by all psychiatric facilities based on a need for safety, as the comment had come on a post discussing involuntary psychiatric admissions. When other commenters responded and noted that they had been searched upon admission to some hospitals but not others, I began to wonder about the necessity of such a practice.

Dialogue is what gives social media its power. If you wonder, you need only to ask. I started with a blog post: 'Tell me your psych unit search stories.' Dozens of comments came in.

The female nurse told me to take off my clothes and I started shaking and sobbing into my hands covering my face. The nurse kept saying, 'Oh, it's no big deal, it's not that bad,' when it clearly was very bad for me. I shook and sobbed and took off my clothes. She said she needed me to take off my underwear, too, and I shook and sobbed and said, 'No no no no no.' She unlatched my bra and took it as far off as possible for a person whose hands are on her face. She pulled my underwear down to my knees. She gave me a gown, which I put on hastily, then I pulled my undergarments back in place. She cheerfully said, 'See, it wasn't that bad!' and left me with a couple blankets and took my clothes and other things. I wrapped myself up in the blankets as tightly as I could, curled up as small as I could, and had a panic attack for the next hour.

People wrote about the humiliation they experienced. They wrote about their beliefs about why body searches were done – for safety, or to document lesions on their skin for the hospital's liability. They talked about the stigma this conveys to psychiatry – that it is not done on medical or surgical units of the hospital even though those patients or their visitors might be dangerous. One reader asked

Can you imagine being admitted to have your gallbladder out and told well it's policy that we have to strip search you because we've had a patient who was violent and another who had substance abuse problems, and someone was smoking in the bathroom on a unit with oxygen tanks, and people will surprise you, and we can never be too careful, and we have to keep other patients and staff safe?

Next, I embedded a survey into our blog in order get an idea of how common a practice this was, at least for our readers who had been hospitalized (Miller, 2012a). The poll was taken by 107 people; 60 had been strip searched while 47 were not. Of the 60 who had been searched, 47 found it to be distressing and 13 did not. While the survey was neither validated nor controlled, and had only a small number of respondents, it was enough to demonstrate that hospitals may vary with regard to search practices, and that patients may vary with response to how they experience events (Miller, 2012b).

Since that time I have learned a trick to increase the circulation (and response numbers) for a poll placed on a blog by cross-linking the poll social media venues including Facebook and Twitter. The link to the survey can be sent out on a Twitter feed with a request to take the poll. While the response rate is likely quite low, I have found that it helps to request a retweet with the simple phrase 'Pls RT', so that the number of people exposed to the poll increases quickly. At times, I have tweeted a direct message (DM) to psychiatrists or advocates with large Twitter followings asking them to tweet a survey link to their followers. On some surveys we have got close to 1000 respondents, even when the surveys have been quite long. The links have been tweeted around the world in a variety of languages. Using social media to gather data on reader attitudes may not be scientifically valid, and the results need to be viewed with caution, but it is both free and fast if the goal is simply to get a sense of whether an issue might warrant further exploration. The idea is not new. A 1998 article (Houston & Fiore, 1998) discussed ways in which Internet surveys could be used, and another study (Klein et al., 2007) looked at smoking rates as determined from online surveys compared with results from national surveys and concluded that online surveys may be useful for public health surveillance.

Finishing up on the strip-search project, I finally resorted to some old-school older forms of communications. I called and emailed people I knew at local psychiatric inpatient hospitals and units, and discovered that the policies for searching patients upon admission varied widely, even in hospitals with similar patient demographics. One hospital did a full visual inspection of the skin (a strip search) while another only asked people to take off their shoes and socks and invert their pockets. Use of metal detector wands was also found to be helpful.

Ultimately, it was not at all clear to me that the needs for safety or liability should differ by hospital, and I concluded that a strip search requirement was unnecessary as blanket policy for psychiatric inpatients. And with that, I wrote an article for *Clinical Psychiatry News*, a publication that is distributed to 40,000 psychiatrists, and titled it, 'It's time to stop strip searching psychiatric patients' (Miller, 2012c).

Does social media make a difference as a means to advocate for better treatment for our patients, and therefore to decrease stigma for both our patients and our profession? It certainly holds as a powerful tool to converse, to query, and ultimately to spread information about what we have learned. The results remain anecdotal and hopefully we will someday be able to discern what the best ways to best understand our patients' needs are and how to most effectively impact our practices.

Closing remarks

Social media are characterized by being more personal, more interactive, and easier to produce than traditional media. Our three 'shrinks' have illustrated their experiences with this interactive, electronic Internet medium, starting with the infancy of this bidirectional communication medium more than 20 years ago and leading up to the current landscape.

One of the common themes across all three personal reflections is that use of social media to extend one's professional range of expression has a very personal effect on how we see our role as psychiatrists. In the same way that addressing the health of 'populations' has become the current focus in healthcare, advocacy and education of the broader public via social media has become mainstream. Where once physicians had to avoid social media or hide their involvement, now healthcare professionals are using social media freely and to great benefit. They are used to teach, train, educate, inform, advocate, connect, and share. All major healthcare institutions, such as the American Medical Association, National Institutes of Health, the Centers for Disease Control, the Institute of Medicine, and the World Health Organization, have embraced blogs, podcasts, Twitter, Facebook, and other forms of social media. The pioneering efforts of innumerable nurses, physicians, psychologists, pharmacists, other healthcare professionals, and patients, have helped to demonstrate the potential and shape what we have today.

Another theme, which is particularly important to psychiatry, is the positive impact of social media on stigma and stereotypes. An Australian study of adolescents using a form of online social media for mental health demonstrated improvements in stigma, understanding, empathy, and help-seeking related to the use of this technology (Burns et al., 2009). A number of social media campaigns have been launched over the past few years as efforts to shine light on the darkness of stigma and stereotypes, including the US Brain and Behavior Research Foundation's ('Know Science. No Stigma'), New York City's National Alliance on Mental Illness (#iwillListen), and the US Department of Defense ('Real Warriors'). By learning about the broad range of experiences of both patients and practitioners, we become much more successful at understanding others. In so doing, we all learn to be more sensitive to different points of view and more understanding of how to apply this awareness in our professional lives.

Mental health professionals and people who possess lived experience with mental health and substance use problems are using social media to educate others about the profession of psychiatry and to advocate for needed change. They use social media to enhance training of future healthcare professionals. And they use social media to advocate for improvements in patient care, in healthcare quality, and in the health-care delivery system. Reflecting on the progress made over the past 20 years, the future seems bright.

Declaration of interest: The authors disclose their obvious interest in the blog, podcast, and book mentioned within. Steve Daviss reports his interest in Fuse Health Strategies LLC and in M3 Information LLC. Annette Hanson and Dinah Miller report no other conflicts of interest. The authors alone are responsible for the content and writing of the paper.

References

Burns, J.M., Durkin, L.A., & Nicholas, J. (2009). Mental health of young people in the United States: What role can the Internet play in reducing stigma and promoting help seeking? *Journal of Adolescent Health, 45*, 95–97.

Daviss, S.R. (1994). SCHIZ-L: Schizophrenia research discussion list. *Retrieved from* http://www.bio.net/mm/neur-sci/1994-February/013298.html

Daviss, S.R. (????) *An Internet Primer for Mental Health Professionals.*

DeJong, S.M., Benjamin, S., Anzia, J.M., John, N., Boland, R.J., Lomax, J., & Rostain, A.L. (2012). Professionalism and the Internet in psychiatry: What to teach and how to teach it. *Academic Psychiatry, 35*(5), 356–362.

Fenwick, T. (2014). Social media and medical professionalism: Rethinking the debate and the way forward. *Academic Medicine, 89*, 1331–1334.

Gitlow, S. (2001). The online community as a healthcare resource. In M.P. Manfredi, B. Bozarth & S. Howell (Eds), *Connecting with the New Healthcare Consumer: Defining Your Strategy.* Jones & Bartlett Learning.

Grande, D., Gollust, S.E., Pany, M., Seymour, J., Goss, A., Kilaru, A., & Meisel, Z. (2014). Translating research for health policy: researchers' perceptions and use of social media. *Health Affairs, 33*(7), 1278–1285.

Greysen, S.R., Kind, T., & Chretien, K.C. (2010). Online professionalism and the mirror of social media. *Journal of General Internal Medicine, 25*(11), 1227–1229.

Houston, J.D., & Fiore, D.C. (1998). Online medical surveys: Using the Internet as a research tool. *MD Computing, 15*(2), 116–120.

Klein, J.D., Thomas, R.K., & Sutter, E.J. (2007). Self-reported smoking in online surveys: Prevalence estimate validity and item format effects. *Medical Care, 45*(7), 691–695.

Lenhart, A., & Fox, S. (2006). *Bloggers.* Pew Research Center Report. *Retrieved from* http://www.pewinternet.org/2006/07/19/bloggers/

Miller, D. (2012a). Strip search survey. Shrink Rap. *Retrieved from* http://psychiatrist-blog.blogspot.com/2012/04/strip-search-poll.html

Miller, D. (2012b). Tell me your psych unit search story. Shrink Rap. *Retrieved from* http://psychiatrist-blog.blogspot.com/2012/04/tell-me-your-psych-unit-search-stories.html

Miller, D. (2012c). It's time to stop strip searching psychiatric patients. *Clinical Psychiatry News Retrieved from* http://www.clinicalpsychiatrynews.com/single-view/it-s-time-to-stop-strip-searching-psychiatric-patients/63bed88d2b1167b9761caf30e9c115b7.html

Miller, D., Hanson, A., & Daviss, S.R. (2011). *Shrink Rap: Three Psychiatrists Explain Their Work.* Baltimore, MD: Johns Hopkins University Press.

Saltzman, J. (2007, May 31). *Blogger unmasked, court case upended. Boston Globe.*

Index

www.ingramcontent.com/pod-product-compliance
Ingram Content Group UK Ltd.
Pitfield, Milton Keynes, MK11 3LW, UK
UKHW012331270225
455677UK00027B/810